音樂氣功

Musical Qigong

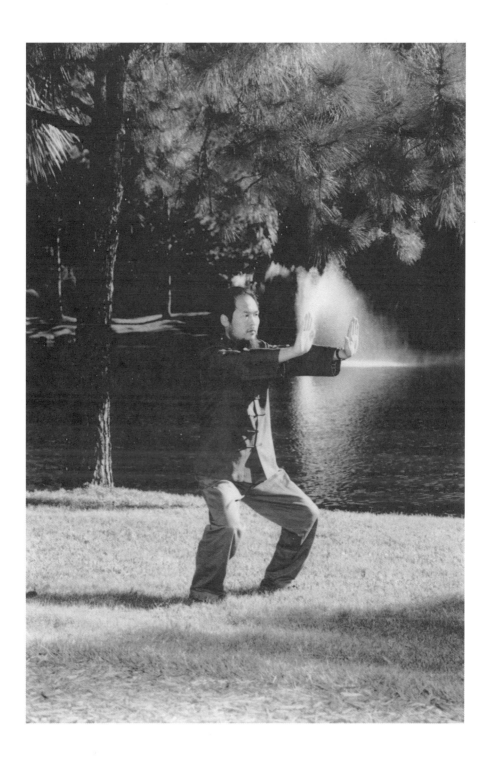

Musical Qigong

Ancient Chinese Healing Art
from a Modern Master

Shen Wu

Illustrated by You Shan Tang

HOMA & SEKEY BOOKS
Dumont, New Jersey

ISBN: 0-9665421-5-0
Library of Congress Card Number: 00-103407

Publishers Cataloging-in-Publication Data
Wu, Shen
Musical Qigong: Ancient Chinese Healing Art from a Modern Master
1. Qigong, Chi kung. 2. Health. 3. Music
I. Title.
RA781.8 .W 2001 613.7/1-dc21

Published by Homa & Sekey Books
138 Veterans Plaza
P. O. Box 103
Dumont, NJ 07628

Tel: (201)384-6692
Fax: (201)384-6055
Email: info@homabooks.com
Website: www.homabooks.com

Editor: Shawn X. Ye
Cover Design: Judy Wang
Illustrator: You Shan Tang

First American Edition

1 3 5 7 9 10 8 6 4 2

For my students and patients

Contents

PART ONE
THEORY OF MUSICAL QIGONG

PART TWO
GENERAL QIGONG EXERCISES

PART THREE
QIGONG EXERCISES FOR THE FIVE ORGANS

PART FOUR
LIFE MUSIC FOR HEALING

PART FIVE
FAQ ABOUT MUSICAL QIGONG

ABOUT THE AUTHOR

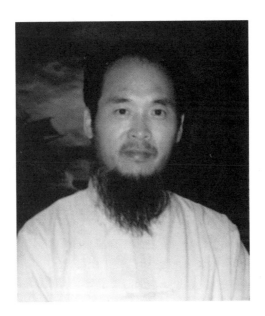

Founder of Musical Qigong and Director of Chinese Traditional Medical Institute, Master Shen Wu is an advanced Qigong practitioner who has devoted his life to teaching Qigong and using Musical Qigong to help others regain their vital life energies. Since mid 1990s, Master Wu has been using Musical Qigong to successfully treat patients, especially those terminal patients who suffer from various kinds of cancer and other diseases.

Master Shen Wu was born into an exceptionally intellectual family with considerable medical background in the city of Shang Qiu, Henan Province, China. His grandfather was a well-known physician who had bestowed the young Shen Wu much of the medical information and the secret treasures of medicine. From an early age, Shen Wu played musical instruments and practiced Qigong. Meanwhile he developed a keen interest in Chinese and Western medicine, ancient literature, music, martial arts and Qigong. Over the years, with the knowledge and medical skills he had obtained from his grandfather and the books the old physician had instructed him to read, Master Wu became very learned, not only in the medical arts of Qigong, herbology, anatomy and physiology, and diagnosis, but also in the arts of calligraphy, philosophy, astrology, and Feng Shui.

A graduate from Henan Chinese Medical School in the late 1970s and a postgraduate in philosophy and political economics from The Superior Official College of Central Government of China in the late 1980s, Master Shen Wu had been a medical Qigong doctor and herbalist in China for over 20 years. Master Wu's work was introduced to the public by many Chinese national media, including China Central Television and New China News Agency.

Since coming to the United States in 1995, Master Shen Wu has lectured and given Musical Qigong treatments in more than ten states. He has appeared, among others, on NBC, CBS and TBS. Master Wu has also been interviewed by such major Chinese media as North American Chinese Television Stations, New York Chinese Television Station and Hong Kong Star Television. Extensive coverage on Master Shen Wu and his Musical Qigong has appeared in the following major newspapers and magazines: World Journal, Orlando Weekly, China Qigong Science, International News, Freedom Times, U.S. Digest and Washington News.

In addition to conducting Musical Qigong classes and offering Musical Qigong treatments to various patients, Master Shen Wu has been working closely with Dr. Neil J. Finkler at Walt Disney Memorial Cancer Institute, and Dr. Thomas J. Katta of Winter Park Memorial Hospital, both traditional medical oncologists in the Orlando area, regarding various treatments for their late stage cancer patients. Master Shen Wu is also co-operating with Dr. Mehmet C. Oz, Assistant Professor of Surgery at Columbia University's College of Physicians & Surgeons, for development on alternative medicine.

In 1999, Master Shen Wu was honored as a "World Famous Traditional Chinese Medical Doctor" by the International Association of Integrated Medicine. In the same year he was recognized as a "World Qigong Master" by International Association of Qigong.

PREFACE

Based on a Speech at Florida Hospital

Commenting on Musical Qigong and the Cancer Trial Program

Three years ago I treated advanced cancer patient Yoko Tominaga. She was operated on and we gave her some chemotherapy about two years ago. A year later, when I was checking some of Yoko's liver enzymes, I saw that some of the enzymes were going up, and some other things were happening. Yoko confessed to me that she had been doing other things. I said, "Yoko, this is really very interesting because you had a cancer and you are well beyond what the normal survival is, but you have no evidence of the disease. I've scanned you six times and all your tumor markers are normal. I never understood. What happened?" Yoko then told me her confession that she had been doing some alternative therapies. She's been taking some herbs, and in addition, she's been doing "Qigong." I said, "What!?" And of course, I've never heard of this before. The subject was dropped for a while.

One day, Yoko's husband Tomi called and said he had a very dear friend (Mrs. Ito) in Japan, who had lung cancer. The doctors had given up; there was nothing they could do. He wanted me to recommend someone she could see. I gave him the name of a medical oncologist to see for her lung cancer. She eventually got intra-bronchial radiation through the windpipe, and she had radiation in the lungs. I spoke with the radiation therapist and medical oncologist. They both told me that we were talking about days at best. They also told me there was no way of her eating again, that her tumor was pressing against her esophagus and she'd be lucky if she could get a sip in. And it has been six to eight weeks before I saw Yoko back in the office, and she said, "You know, it's an amazing thing. Not only is she alive but she has no pain, which was a big component. She was eating, breathing, and she was feeling a lot better." I was very skeptical at the time.

A few days later Tomi asked me if I would like to see one of these Qigong therapies. I had to see what this Qigong therapy was all about. So I went down to Tomi's house and actually witnessed treatment for this patient with end-stage lung cancer, which conventional medicine had given up on. I brought my wife with me, and that was the first time I ever actually met Master Wu. As we sat in that room, certain things were happening. After we left Tomi's house, my wife looked at me and said, "It got so cold in that room. It was freezing! When we first walked into that room, it was really very warm." My wife said that she saw the thermostat on the wall and nobody was touching it. On subsequent visit, Master Wu explained to me what happened in the room and the principles behind all that. After a few more visits, we decided we were going to embark on a little trial. The trial was going to be on patients of mine, that I know that conventional medicine really had nothing more to offer.

Several things became very apparent about Qigong therapy. One, it certainly doesn't hurt anybody. And probably the easiest thing for Qigong to do is to take pain away. One of my patients, a woman in her thirties or forties with end-stage cervical cancer, had severe, severe pain. She came in with kidney failure. She had failed radiation therapy and chemotherapy. We decided we weren't going to perform any more therapies. I spoke to the family and said I had nothing more to offer. I also asked if they would like to have Master Wu come. We talked a bit and surely Master Wu came. The patient was bed-ridden for days and was on high doses of morphine for pain relief by IV. About an hour after the first treatment, I received a call from the nurse. The nurse said the patient wanted her pain medication decreased because she was not having any pain. I said sure. In the morning when I visited the patient who was on pain medication for weeks, she was now completely off morphine. From that point on, she was completely off morphine. She started to drink, eat, and asked to get out of the bed. Her kidney problem also started to turn around. She began to make urine.

Of the group of patients that we have looked at, there is no question in my mind that Master Wu's treatment has led to a prolongation of quality life, as these people lived much longer than I had ever expected. And they lived a life that is pain free. I am very interested in Qigong therapy and, as you may know about, the National Cancer Institute is also very interested and now has a branch for the investigation of alternative medicine and therapies.

There are really a lot of alternative treatments that are fake, hocus-pocus, and money making opportunities that only take advantage of people, and they do absolutely nothing. But there's no doubt in my mind that Master Wu is of the utmost sincerity in what he does.

Neil J. Finkler, M.D.
Gynecologic Oncology Cancer Specialist
Walt Disney Memorial Cancer Institute Florida Hospital
Assistant Professor of Gynecology at Harvard Medical School
Division Director of Gynecologic Oncology at Boston University Medical Center

FOREWORD

For a long time, the majority of the people in the Western world thought of the human being in tripartite terms—made up of body, mind and spirit. The care of the body was consigned to the medical establishment; the mind was the purview of the educational system; and the spirit came under the domain of religious institutions.

But, during the upheavals of the 1960s, when body, mind and spirit all seemed to merge into a psychedelic blur, Westerners began to look at life differently. We asked questions and expanded our understanding. We began to look to the East, where humans were thought of more as a blended *whole*, a unity of body-mind-spirit, for answers. Words like "holistic" entered the common vocabulary. The concepts of *yin* and *yang* lost their mystery. The medical world was assaulted by individuals seeking an enhanced quality of life. They came with ideas of "prevention" and "alternative therapies" on their lips. They began to find healers who practiced acupuncture, herbal remedies and healing touch. People noticed that something fundamental was missing from education. Many sought Gurus in the search for enlightenment. The Wisdom of the Ancients crept into the headlines of today.

As physicists reported on discoveries about energy fields and it became apparent that the human body was not unlike the entire universe in its energy make-up, the ancient Chinese concept of Qi (energy) and the energy meridians (energy channels) of the body no longer seemed mythical. American doctors made pilgrimages to China to study the effects of acupuncture for anesthesia and pain control. Health food stores were overrun with requests for an ever widening variety of Chinese herbal products. Television programs featured demonstrations of graceful movements with strange-sounding names like "tai chi" and "Qigong." How amazing, we thought, that all this information was thousands of years old. Where had we been that we were just now hearing of it? I, like many others, opened my mind to explore this new/old thought.

In the midst of this evolution of Western thinking, Shen Wu was born in China into a family steeped in Chinese medical culture. As he grew older, he gave his body to the practice of Qigong exercises, his mind to education in health and healing and his spirit to the inspiration of the Divine. His healing music flowed from his inner connection with that Divine Spirit. He became a unified body-mind-spirit entity—healer, musician, teacher, humanitarian and spiritual guide—in short, a Master.

I met Master Shen Wu and was introduced to his Musical Qigong therapy shortly after a major life crisis. My doctor had just said to me, "Your biopsy shows that you have endometrial cancer."

The serendipitous events that led from that diagnosis to a state of complete health took me down an amazing path. It began when I accidentally heard about Qigong while attending a professional seminar in my field of psychotherapy. I subsequently watched a video describing Master Wu's Musical Qigong which contained a testimonial regarding the efficacy of Qigong for improving quality of life and ending the pain of terminal cancer patients. What was my surprise when I recognized the physician on the video, Dr. Neil Finkler, as the one gynecological oncologist that had been recommended to me by four out of four doctors! As he contemplated what he had witnessed with Master Wu, he allowed himself to wonder aloud about what Master Wu might do for people who came to him earlier in their illnesses. I decided there and then that I would avail myself of the healing qualities of Master Wu's Musical Qigong *before* I became a "terminal patient."

As I experienced a Musical Qigong therapy session with Master Wu, I was filled with such a glorious feeling of love and light, balance and harmony that I immediately knew I would follow his recommendation and complete twenty such sessions before going into surgery. My surgeon, Dr. Finkler, agreed to do a second biopsy at the end of the treatments.

During the six weeks from my first to last Musical Qigong sessions, I began to learn Qigong exercises, performing them daily to Master's Wu's music, which is based on the Chinese five-tone musical scale corresponding to the five organs identified by ancient men of medicine. I also began to study the theory and principles of Shen Wu's Musical Qigong, as well as the philosophy behind the exercises. In the course of therapy sessions I experienced visions of moving colors, energized *yin* and *yang* symbols and piercing shafts of light coming through an open door and entering my body. My energy increased and my state of health became vibrant. My friends and associates all commented on my energy and spirit, saying I appeared "radiant." I felt absolutely no fear regarding my condition, but instead, a calm inner awareness that all was well.

My second biopsy, after the twenty Qigong treatments, still showed some cancer remaining in the lining of my uterus, and surgery was scheduled. The surgery was quick and easy. I recovered rapidly, feeling well enough to return to work after two weeks. Pathology reports indicated that the cancer "was confined to the inner one-third of the uterine wall, 2.4 mm maximum thickness, 1 mm maximum depth of invasion into inner one-third of myometrium. No lymphovascular invasion is identified." No malignancy was found in the ovaries, tubes, lymph nodes, pelvic washings or diaphragm washings. All was clean and clear, no cancer remaining. My doctors proclaimed me "cured."

It is my knowing that my experience with Qigong and its energy balancing effects allowed my body to reduce the virulence of the cancer and to release the disease process from surrounding tissue. I continue to feel vibrant and radiant, embracing life in all its aspects.

It is with great joy and honor that I write this "Foreword" to Master Shen Wu's book on Musical Qigong. I know that anyone seeking to release a disease process, to obtain a greater understanding of the meaning of life, to learn relaxation from physical and mental tension, to achieve a more focused intelligence and a deepening awareness of spirit will find truth and comfort in the words of this book. But it is the practice of the principles that uplifts and inspires.

The ever-turning wheel of life with its balance, harmony and oneness is especially evident to me as I contemplate a portion of my ancestral history which I reported to Master Wu: "Five generations ago, my great-great-grandfather left Midway, Georgia, to journey to China as a missionary from the Presbyterian Church, U.S. Five generations later, a man from China is a missionary to me."

May all who come in contact with this book and with Master Shen Wu's Musical Qigong therapy be blessed, as I feel I have been blessed, with radiant health of body, mind and spirit.

Gini W. Cucuel, M.S.
Licensed Mental Health Counselor
Licensed Marriage and Family Therapist

PART ONE

THEORY OF
MUSICAL QIGONG

A precious component of the Chinese culture and an important part of Chinese healing art, Qigong dates back thousands of years in the Chinese civilization. Music, while primarily the luxury of the royal and noble families in ancient China, was used together with Qigong to treat patients. Unfortunately, this form of therapy had fallen into disuse by and large for political reasons in China. Through more than twenty years of medical Qigong practice and research in both China and the United States, I have "rediscovered" these two ancient Chinese healing arts and combined them together to form a unique way for contemporary healing called "Shen Wu's Musical Qigong" or "Dong Fang Fu Yin Gong" in Chinese.

What I intend to do in this book is explain what Musical Qigong is, how we perform it and why we can benefit from practicing it.

1

Qigong as a Therapy

In recent years, Westerners have become more familiar with acupuncture treatment, a Chinese way of curing disease and physical problems by placing acupuncture needles on the patient's acupoints, locations where the Qi and blood of the internal organs gather and collect. In Chinese, Qi means energy and Gong stands for skill or exercise.

Qigong is a more advanced technique than acupuncture, and does not involve the mechanical application of needles. Qigong is based on a series of exercises that increase the flow of vital energy in the body by stimulating and balancing the flow of the Qi meridians. Meridians are channels or pathways for the movement of Qi within the human body that connect internal organs to other parts of the body. Like an electrical circuit, if the body's energy does not flow freely, the body does not function properly. By increasing the body's flow of inner energy, it is able to fight disease and help heal itself, enabling the body to

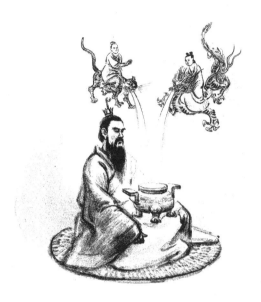

Ming Dynasty Taoist Priest Zhang Sanfeng,
an advocate of Qigong therapy

fight viruses and heal torn muscles, for example.

Qigong is instrumental to maintaining our health and increasing our energy for daily living. Serious practitioners report an abundance of energy, less need for sleep to feel refreshed, and more resistance to colds and flu and other ordinary maladies. They also report a substantial reduction in their day-to-day stress levels. Everyone now recognizes the importance of stress reduction in healthcare.

In addition to maintaining health and energy, work is being done with Qigong and cancer patients. Advanced practitioners of Qigong use Qigong to treat cancer patients, sharing their energy to help their patients regain their own vital life energy, much like a fully charged battery that can recharge a discharged battery by a "jump start." The patients' own bodies can help heal themselves with increased inner energy.

2

Energy Transfer in Musical Qigong

Musical Qigong is a special healing energy therapy that combines two ancient Chinese traditions—healing music and Qigong. In Musical Qigong the ancient Chinese healing music is recorded with modern musical technology to incorporate sound waves with Qigong energy.

Musical Qigong enlivens the mind, relaxes the body and lifts the spirit. It also enhances one's energy and opens the potential power of the human mind. While music is a special language between people and nature, connecting the individual—body, mind and spirit—to the universe, Musical Qigong is a cultural gift to all those who seek to better their health conditions.

A necessary condition for the transmission and reception of energy healing and physical and mental enhancement is an open and honest heart. This applies to both the teacher and the student. A martial art concept that says "you can teach by mouth . . . but you transmit knowledge by heart" implies that the open heart of the student is able to receive the soul and spiritual energy from the teacher. The Qigong master "transfers the energy by heart" to the student, passing his strong bio energy magnetic field onto the student's weak magnetic field. Transmitting knowledge "by heart" has been the traditional Chinese way, generation after generation.

Musical Qigong embodies the same concept. Embedded within the music are messages, which include the energy of Qigong culture, Chinese medical culture and Chinese musical culture. In all types of Qigong practice and therapy the method must be learned from the master, but the student must practice to gain his or her own energy.

There is an ancient Chinese saying: "Honest heart . . . Miracle happens." If one practices with an honest heart, the message and energy will be received in some form—light, electricity, heat, wave energy, magnetic energy or sound. When the student feels heat, cold or numbness inside the palms of the hands, he or she is connected.

The healing energy experienced by patients who seek my Musical Qigong treatments comes from the secret of transmitting by heart. I send my strong energy (energy of the heart) to the patient, who feels better immediately as the immune system is enhanced. The only requirements for receiving this energy are a relaxed body and an open heart. Under these conditions the channels of the body will be open and the energy will flow freely.

Musical Qigong is relatively easy for the beginner and there are no negative side effects. Rather, the music brings balance to mind and body, improving the function of the immune system and prolonging life.

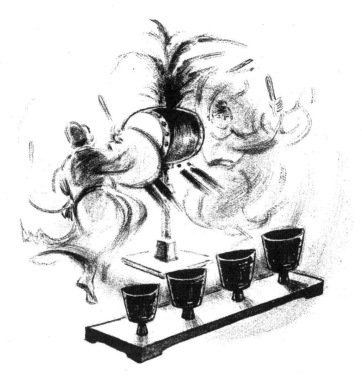

Drum therapy in Anciet China

Students from all walks of life are welcome to experience Musical Qigong. Each person can progress at his or her own pace. The old Chinese saying "There is no earlier or later once you get into the door; there is no higher or lower once you get the wisdom" suggests that age, talent, ability and level of learning are unimportant. All will get the wisdom if the practice is consistent. Musical Qigong enhances life activities and practices regardless of a person's background or religion. The saying "Do it better with music" reflects a global understanding. Henry Wadsworth Longfellow said, "Music is the universal language of mankind," indicating that it cuts across all boundaries and barriers.

The effective practice of Qigong requires the student to put thoughts and worries aside, letting the mind be empty. When connecting to the energy from the universe, one must be calm and quiet, having an attitude of openness, humbleness and respect. Respect for one's teacher translates into respect for oneself. From this perspective the student receives bountiful energy through the teacher and from the universe in a fashion similar to using a television—turn on the power, switch to the right channel and receive signals via the antenna.

By the same token, even when the student is reading about Musical Qigong, his or her body should be relaxed and the mind should observe the palms of the hand and the relationship between the palms and the inside and outside of the body. After a while, the reader may experience the message and energy from Musical Qigong. Sensations may arise between the eyebrows. The palms may feel sore, numb, cold or hot. There may be feelings of pressure, vibrations, and pulsating or penetrating reactions. The lower abdomen may seem warm.

Musical Qigong is especially beneficial to those who are students of other Qigong practices because it increases the possibility of feeling the energy.

3

Music and Medicine: Words and Their Stories

森 **+** 一 **=** 藥
MUSIC + HERB = MEDICINE

A Chinese character is composed of the form and the meaning. However, people seldom notice the composition of the character for "medicine." The symbol for "herb" is on the top and the symbol for music, on the bottom. Further, the character for "music" is composed of three words—"white," "wood," and "silk," respectively. In ancient times, these were all musical instruments. The ancient Chinese believed in the five elements—metal, wood, water, fire and earth—which were held to compose the physical universe and were later used in traditional Chinese medicine to explain various physiological phenomena. According to the five elements, the white color corresponds to metal. It is the symbol for the lung, which takes air into the body (inspiration), and where the spirit is said to reside. Wood is the symbol for the liver, which corresponds to the circulation of blood. The ancient Chinese associated the liver with the soul, for they believed that the soul was lodged in the liver.

Tradition has it that the combination of the soul and the spirit results in strong circulation and well being, allowing for the emergence of blood enlightenment.

A closer look at the character "music" reveals that on the top of the character there are two characters for "silk" sandwiching the character "white." Music played with the silk (string) instrument can touch the heart and soothe the heart meridian (energy channel). Also, music strengthens the heart and keeps the spirit and the soul circulating throughout the body. One, having recovered from illness, would express joy. That is why, in Chinese, the character for "music" also means "joy."

Music = White + Wood + Silk

樂 ＝ 白 ＋ 木 ＋ 絲

As time passed, people discovered that herbs could be useful in treating physical ailments. They then added "herb" to the top of the character for "music," completing the word for "medicine." With the increase in efficacy of herbal medicine, the use of music as medicine had by and large vanished.

Politics also played a role in the disappearance of music as medical treatment. Music became popular in the beginning of Spring and Autumn period (about 722-484 BC). The ruling classes, however, feared that people were so intoxicated with music that the military forces would be weakened and the country would become defenseless. Therefore, they ruled that mu-

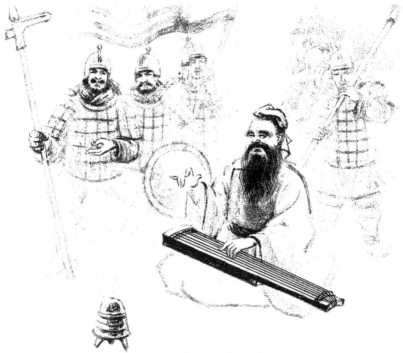

Confucius playing qin,
a seven-stringed plucked instrument similar to the zither

sic could only be played in the palace. Subsequently, Confucius decided to rate music, dictating what could be listened to in accordance with one's social status. During the Qin Dynasty (221-206 BC), the emperor burned almost all books and buried many scholars alive. All the musical scores were burned and music as a medical treatment disappeared. Though recollected in the Tang Dynasty (618-907), music as medical treatment was only permitted for the royal families. The rulers of the Song Dynasty (960-1279) regarded music as an extravagant way of life, thus rendering it unpopular.

4

The Research into
Musical Therapy

The earliest music mankind enjoyed came from nature
– the birds chirping, the insects humming, the wind
hissing, and the water dribbling. According to ancient
Chinese medical literature, the sound of nature and the human
body has a very close relationship. *The Yellow Emperor's Internal Classics,* the "bible of the ancient Chinese medicine," states:
"Up in the sky there are five notes. In the human body there
are five [*yin*] organs … There is a correspondence between the
human body and the sky and earth." It also asserts: "The way
of nature (one of which is sound) cultivates what lives in nature." *Categories of Sutra,* an important medical writing from
the Ming Dynasty (1368-1644), maintains: "Music is the harmonious Qi of the sky and the earth … One hears melody, and
in the process of harmonizing sound with melody, music is
created." This idea suggests that the source of music originates
from the sounds of nature.

This sound of nature has a positive effect on the health of a human body. For example, people with gastro-enteric indigestion can listen to music for recovery. Research so far has proven that music can increase the gastro-enteric peristalsis and promote the secretion of saliva. Most people have experienced a time of fatigue, which might be described as being "brain dead." Listening to a passage of music that comes from nature quickly alleviates this problem. For some people, insomnia is untreatable by medicine. However, if they listen to a passage of rain sound before going to bed, they fall asleep easily. Rumor has it that Marshal Lin Biao, Chairman Mao Zedong's defense minister, had his bed installed with a device that mimicked the sound of rain.

The sound of nature under special circumstances has the ultimate power of communicating beyond the living and the dead. According to ancient literature, there was an infant boy who had a summer stroke with "wind shock" (a Chinese medical term). His breathing was very weak and he was about to die. At that time, the diagnosis was that "wind pathogenic factor has entered and was trapped within the heart meridian. Only when the meridian opened up would the infant survive" (again, this is according to the diagnosis model and theories of Chinese medicine). However, all attempts to revive him failed and he was left dead in an open field. Suddenly, "GONG-GONG-GONG," the thunder broke out and rocked the infant boy on the open ground. He immediately started crying, and the rescuers realized that he was alive again. They came forward to pick him up but the boy was able to walk by himself. Everyone there was shocked and speechless. They wondered if the sound of thunder could treat illnesses too. Yes, they were right. It was the sound of thunder that opened up the stagnation of Qi in his heart meridian.

This example illustrates that music from nature definitely has healing power. Later on, people imitated this in order to

33

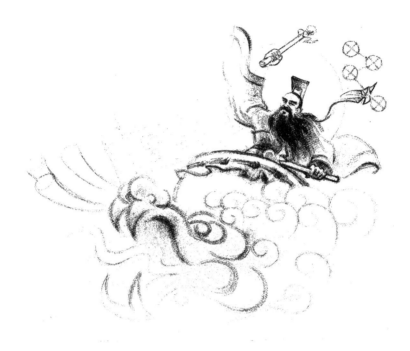

*Yellow Emperor, a legendary ruler in prehistoric period,
synonymous with the father of Chinese civilization*

treat illnesses. A general's wife had a mysterious disease and no doctors or medicine could cure her. Finally a physician said to the general, "Her heart has accumulated heat and the condition is not treatable by any herbs. You should use mind treatment technique and hit the marching drums." The general then had someone beating the drums vigorously in the presence of his wife. Miraculously his wife was healed. Also, for patients with trapped measles that wouldn't come out, doctors ignited firework sticks to scare and shock the patients and the measles came out.

5

Balancing
Yin and Yang

The Chinese word "Yi" or "I" (as in *I-Ching*) is made up of two characters: the sun and the moon — the combination of *yin* and *yang*. It means change, as in *The Book of Change* (*I-Ching*).

The philosophy of *yin-yang* maintains that the material world is the result of the rivalry and unification of the *yin* Qi (energy) and *yang* Qi. Rivalry perceives *yin-yang* as the division of one into two while unification recognizes *yin-yang* as the combination of two into one. Nature is a unified entity which combines with human beings to form the whole entity of *yin-yang* and taiji (tai-chi). In the eyes of a *yin-yang* philosopher, when a person is sick, it is because he or she has a *yin-yang* imbalance.

Music regulates the *yin-yang* balance of a human being with its sound wave (a form of energy). The human body has certain physiological rhythms. These rhythms can be superimposed by musical rhythms, resulting in a resonance effect. If someone gets sick because of an external *yin-yang* Qi imbalance, he or she can use music to regulate such imbalance. Through the vibratory frequency of its sound wave, musical energy can induce a resonance effect with the internal physiological rhythmic activities of the human body, influencing and rectifying the unbalanced condition. This is called musical therapy for *yin-yang* imbalance.

When someone has a decrease in bodily functioning or is emotionally depressed, his or her internal *yin-yang* balance is upset. According to the theory of "Increase *Yang* for *Yin* diseases," one should adopt therapeutic music for *yin* type diseases to help promote the rise of *yang* Qi in the body. The music stimulates the functionality of body mechanisms and uplifts emotions, thereby returning the body to a state of *yin-yang* balance. For example, if one has depression, one can listen to *Gong*-type music, which is usually a lively and uplifting rhythm.

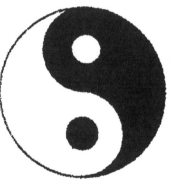

Chinese medicine views the relationship between musical therapy and the human body as that of unification between time and space. An example of the relationship comes from the tai-chi *yin-yang* revolution, or rotation. The noted Ming Dynasty medical scholar Zhang Jing Yue (1563-1640) once said, "Tai-chi is quiescent and dynamic and it has *yin* and *yang*. Therefore, heaven and earth are quiescent and dynamic. Quiescence and dynamics are the *yin-yang*." The human body responds to musical therapy by correcting the circular revolution of the internal *yin-yang*, causing it to adjust to the external *yin-yang* of nature. When there is a balance between the internal and external *yin-yang* rotation, diseases will be gone.

6

Musical Therapy
and the Heart

From Chinese medicine we learn that the "heart governs mental and spiritual clarity and brilliance." The heart is also seen as the source for the seven complex emotional states—happiness, anger, worry, pensiveness, sadness, fear and shock. Therefore, we can say that "emotions are all manipulated by the heart." Musical therapy primarily affects the heart-mind-spirit.

The Yellow Emperor's Internal Classics stated: "Heart contains the spirit. If the spirit is not contained, the body is not healthy." Wu Shang Xian, a prominent Qing Dynasty (1644-1911) doctor, wrote in *External Treatment Medical Discussion*: "For illnesses originating from the seven emotions, looking at flowers to reduce boredom and listening to songs to reduce sadness are better than taking herbs." Therefore, these emotional illnesses can be treated with entertainment therapies targeted at

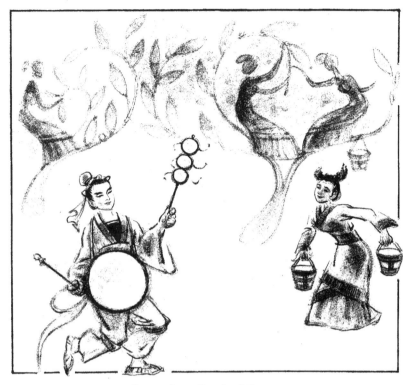

Scene from Book of Songs,
one of the four greatest Chinese classics

the heart.

When the emotional states are functioning normally, they are under the control of the heart-mind-spirit. When they become disturbed and turn into abnormal states, they first affect the related organ, then the body and limbs. In treating the root cause of the disturbance, musical therapy can be administered to the heart, bringing recovery under certain conditions. Chinese medicine assigns to the heart the role of governing the blood vessels. Because musical therapy promotes blood and Qi circulation, the heart-mind-spirit can be effectively nurtured.

7

Music Promotes Immunity

Contemporary science provides an understanding of how music can treat illnesses. The human body is made up of several systems that coordinate their functions in orderly rhythmic movements or vibrations. Brain wave activity, heartbeat, the expansion and contraction of the lungs, gastrointestinal peristalsis, and the autonomic nervous system all have rhythmic movements. When music of a certain frequency matches that of an internal system or organ, resonance occurs and creates a pleasant sensation both physically and psychologically. The most suitable frequency for human sensation is about 70-90 vibrations per minute, which is close to the heart rate.

When a person is sick, each of the affected systems will have a different vibrational rhythm. The healing music should be chosen according to its specific harmonious pitch vibration in order to return each system to its normal and even optimal vibrational frequency, promoting recovery of the patient. Here is a story of a female scientist whose experiences can prove this theory. For a while after she got home from work, the scientist always felt tense and grumpy. One night, she heard her daughter playing some fast beat disco music and felt that the music, matching her mood, was able to make her calmer and more relaxed. In fact, this scientist had found a suitable music type for the initial stage of her musical therapy. In musical therapy, at the beginning, one can use music that matches his or her mood. Then, he or she can modify the music gradually to match certain desirable emotional states.

Research has shown that music, comprised of seven tones with an orderly sound wave vibration with a frequency at around 35Hz, produces certain energy which, after entering the body, carries out a harmonious resonance with body cells. There is a massage effect on the cells.

Music can also regulate the internal atmosphere of the human body, promote the activities of the endocrine system, and enhance metabolism. In addition, music can increase the degree of excitement of the cerebral cortex and induce corresponding activities of the central nervous system. It can calm emotions, alleviate nervous conditions, and regulate the function of all bodily systems, thereby assisting people to recover from fatigue, regain energy, and increase immunity.

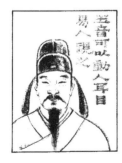
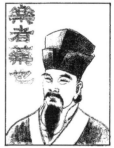

*Doctors who advocated
musical therapy*

*Zhang Zihe   Zhu Danxi
(1156-1228)   (1281-1358)*

8

Music Promotes Brain Balance and Creativity

Specialists worldwide have noted that music has the ability to open up and develop the potential of the left and right hemispheres of the brain as well as balance their functioning.

The human brain has two large cerebral hemispheres of basically the same structure. They are linked by a thick band of nerve fibers, the corpus callosum. Some higher activities such as speech and writing are controlled from one cerebral hemisphere, the dominant one and usually the left hemisphere. It is also called the "speech brain." The non-dominant side is important in visual-spatial orientation and may be involved in artistic appreciation and creative thought. This is also called the "music brain."

In everyday life, mankind cannot do away with speech. Because the "speech brain" (the left hemisphere) is constantly being utilized and developed, the right hemisphere is relatively less used and underdeveloped. This results in the functional imbalance of the left and right brains. We know that although the left brain can deal with logical knowledge in detail, it has a hard time seeing the big picture to make judgments about wholes or developing artistic experience and geometric visualization. The right brain comes to the rescue. It is good at creativity, association, objectivity, and intuition. If both hemispheres can be evenly developed and utilized, it will be a big leap forward for mankind's intelligence.

So how to develop the right brain, the artistic or "music brain?" In music itself, we find the answer.

While using the "speech brain" extensively for working and learning, a person can help activate new excitement areas on the right brain by taking time out to appreciate music, giving the "speech brain" space for rest and restoration. Moreover, it can relieve the condition of imbalance resulting from one brain hemisphere being in the suppressive mode for an extended period of time, increase the excitement level on the cerebral cortex, and correspondingly increase the capability of neural transmission and memory storage, allowing a fuller development of both sides of the brain. As psychologist Lou Lawrence once said: "Only when the right brain is also sufficiently utilized will a person be most creative."

The great physicist Albert Einstein enjoyed physics and music throughout his life. In order to produce his great work, he needed the effective functioning of both his extremely logical and inductive left brain and his highly image-oriented and imaginative right brain. In 1985 Dr. Marian Diamond of University of California at Berkeley found that Einstein's brain had four times more 'oligodendroglia'—helper cells that speed neural communication—than the brains of eleven gifted people she also studied. We can speculate that his love of music and his enjoy-

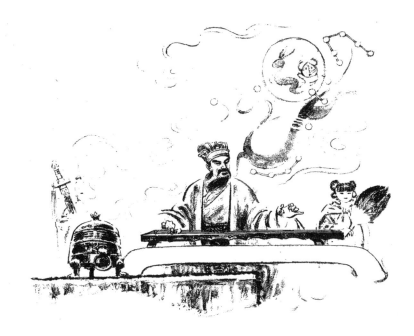

Military strategist Zhuge Liang (181-234)

ment in performing may have contributed to this phenomenon.

In China, the use of music to promote intellectual activities has a very long history. *The Book of Old Tang: Scroll 190* stated: "Emperor Pu asked for music. Each time his train of thought slowed down, he would play music. When his mind was energized, he would compose essays."

During the Spring and Autumn period, Confucius highly recommended the use of music. His disciple wrote the *Book of Rites* to record his sayings and activities. Music was discussed in many chapters.

In today's world of information, what is the most precious thing? It is not gold. It is not physical assets. It is human intelligence, which consists primarily of five basic components—memory, observation, attention, imagination, and cognition.

When there is a problem with one of these components, the quality of a person's overall intelligence is affected, as well as the functioning of the other four components. For example, a low level of memory can bring down the level of observation, attention, imagination, and cognition.

The potential of human intelligence far surpasses current human experience. The brain contains 140 to 160 billion highly specialized nerve cells. Contemporary research identifies a storage capacity for the memory of messages in the brain of a normal individual as between 10^{12} to 10^{15} bytes, about 1 million times bigger than that of an electronic calculator. It is equivalent to the total information capacity of all the libraries in the world.

There may be many ways to improve memory and develop intelligence, and using music to do so may bring miraculous results. Just as Einstein once said: "From music, I got my inspirations for many of my scientific achievements."

Physiologically speaking, music can induce the body to secret beneficial hormones responsible for regulating blood circulation, neural cell excitement level, and memory processes. In short, music enhances intelligence.

9

Music Is the
Lubricant of Life

Music is the lubricant of life. Although the number of tones is limited, wonderful melodies and amazing effects can be produced. Clinicians have discovered that the blood pressure of hypertensive patients decreased after listening to violin music; the pain of women in labor was reduced as they listened to melodious music while giving birth; stuttering patients had a faster rate of recovery when practicing singing; and patients with neural disease felt fewer symptoms when they heard soothing music. In fact, musical therapy is being used frequently now as an adjunct to traditional medical treatment. It has truly become the lubricant of life.

Life on the contemporary scene is becoming more stressful and chaotic, providing a breeding ground for many physical and psychological diseases. Medical experts recognize that over-

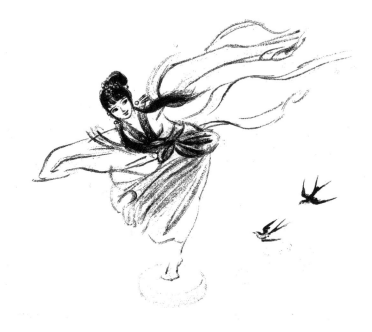

Flying Sparrow (Feiyan) Zhao (? - 1 BC)
a Han Dynasty singer and dancer, later an empress

extended people would benefit from selecting, appreciating, singing and playing music for the enjoyment such activity brings,
as well as the healing and soothing effects on the body. Music
effectively relaxes the body mechanism and facilitates coping
with life circumstances, thereby promoting health and longevity.

10

The Five-Note
Guidance Theory

The treatment principles for Musical Qigong are based on the Five-Note Guidance Theory. The word Guidance came from Zhuang-zi's *Determinant*: "Guiding emotions to harmony. Guiding body to relaxation." It means that through the use of music, the listener is guided to an optimal state where the whole body, including all joints and tendons, is relaxed and the heart and mind harmoniously regulated."

The Five-Note Guidance Theory has its roots in the ancient mathematical models used by traditional Chinese music *The River Diagram* and *The Book of Music*. It also has close relationship with the physiological rhythm of the human body.

Naturally, the Five-Note Guidance Theory has to do with the five notes. Unlike modern music, the ancient Chinese music system was composed of five notes. These five notes are

Gong, Shang, Jue, Zhi, and *Yu,* corresponding, respectively, to the five elements—metal, wood, water, fire and earth. They also respond to the five internal organs—spleen, lungs, liver, heart, and kidneys. Further, they relate to the five tastes—bitter, salty, sweet, sour, and spicy.

YU

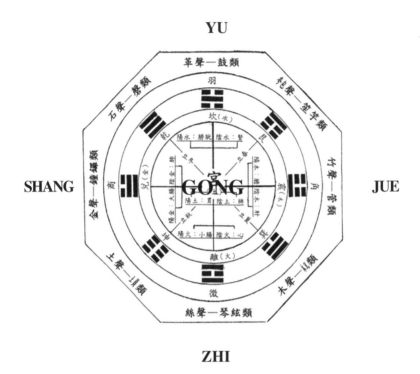

SHANG   **GONG**   **JUE**

ZHI

- ◆ Gong—Earth—Spleen—Bitter
- ◆ Shang—Metal—Lungs—Salty
- ◆ Jue—Wood—Liver—Sweet
- ◆ Zhi—Fire—Heart—Sour
- ◆ Yu—Water—Kidneys—Spicy

Gong type guidance music has *Gong* sound as the primary note. According to Chinese medicine, *Gong* note belongs to the earth type and relates to the spleen and stomach. Its character is mediating and mild. The spleen "stores" the mind of ideas and cognitive thoughts. Its emotion characteristics are pensive, quiet and soft, classic and elegant. Its sound is extremely loud, downward, and cloudy. *Gong* type music can promote the function of the spleen and stomach.

Shang type guidance music has *Shang* sound as the primary note. The *Shang* note belongs to the metal type and relates to the lungs and large intestine. Its character is cleansing and clearing. The lung "stores" the *yang*-spirit. It helps maintain normal water metabolism. Its emotion characteristic is melancholy. Its sound is high octave, melodious, and downhearted. Its feeling of cleansing and quietness can help improve the breathing rhythm.

Jue type guidance music has *Jue* sound as the primary note. The *Jue* note belongs to the wood type and relates to the liver and gallbladder. Its character is barrier-less extension. The liver "stores" the *yin*-spirit. It has the function of smoothing and regulating the flow of Qi and blood. Its emotion characteristic is anger. Its sound is smooth, soft, free flowing, and soothing.

Zhi type guidance music has *Zhi* sound as the primary note. The *Zhi* note belongs to the fire type and relates to the heart and small intestine. Its character is brightening and expanding. The heart "stores" the mind-spirit and governs mental activities. Its emotion characteristic is happiness. Its sound is strong, exciting, active, and lively. It helps promote the metabolic functionality of the human body.

Yu type guidance music has *Yu* sound as the primary note. The *Yu* note belongs to the water type and relates to the kidneys and urinary bladder. Its character is flowing and running wild. The kidneys "store" determination and govern growth and development of the body. Its emotion characteristic is fright, opening wide, running wild, as well as mournful. Its sound is

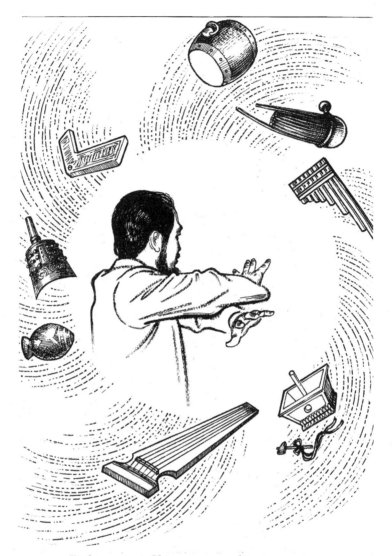

Eight ancient Chinese musical instruments

extremely short, high, sharp and clear. It helps strengthen the kidneys and bones and promotes the production of essence and bone marrow. As a result, *Yu* type guidance music energizes mental activities, promoting a quicker mind and a better memory as well as improving the hearing capacity.

11

Fundamental Principles of Musical Qigong

Based on the Five-Note Guidance Theory, the music in my Qigong therapy consists of five pentatonic tones that correspond to the five major organs of the body: the liver, the heart, the spleen, the lungs and the kidneys. Sound waves, known as mechanical waves, serve as an electrical medium, stimulating the organs in the body through acupuncture points. Music, therefore, enhances circulation of the blood, balances the energy systems and restores the health of the body. The resonance between the musical sound wave and the bodily cells promotes the regulation of the bodily Qi and blood, which in turn promotes the immune system and the function of internal organs.

With the help of electronic musical synthesizers, I have produced soothing healing Qigong music with Chinese styled melodies to accompany my patient treatment. While treating patients, I deliver positive Qi to them through the universal energy. This energy has been found to stimulate the internal organs and open the meridians and acupuncture points, resulting in improved blood circulation, immunity, body strength and good health. In cancer patients it has restrained the growth of cancer cells, decreased inflammation and blood loss, relieved pain and prolonged life.

Qigong works under the assumption that there are both good and bad energies in the body. Qigong teaches a person to direct the positive energy into the body and to direct the negative energy out of the body. The more proficient one becomes at directing the different types of energy to enhance the good energy, the healthier one becomes.

Philosophy, morality, and spirituality all work hand-in-hand with the physical principles of Qigong to enhance a person's general health by maintaining a healthy mind and soul.

So how can we attain to all this? The following are the principles a Qigong student must observe.

MORALLY VIRTUOUS

The Yellow Emperor, the educator Confucius, and the philosopher Lao-zi were some of the pioneering practitioners of Qigong. They all believed that in order to be a successful practitioner of Qigong one must have a good heart and be morally virtuous. A Qigong practitioner has to perform good deeds. The more selfless the practitioner becomes, the greater his or her own energy is enhanced. The mind will be calm, and the heart will be virtuous—a necessary preparation for practicing Qigong. For those who perform bad deeds or are selfish, the energy will not flow properly in the body. Thus, the Qigong practitioner must always perform good deeds in order to maintain good energy.

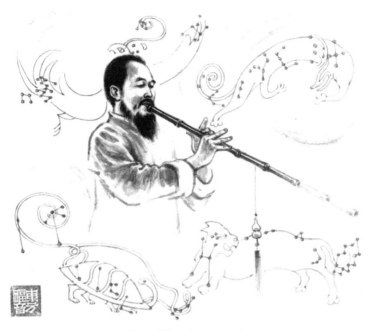

Shen Wu playing xiao
(a vertical bamboo flute)

THE TEACHER

Finding a good teacher is fundamental. There are many secrets and methods of Qigong that can only be learned from a good teacher. Even if one is born with an innate ability to practice Qigong and practices the principles and exercises rigorously, the art cannot be mastered without proper tutelage.

When looking for a teacher, keep in mind that his or her good moral and philosophical standing is more important than his or her popularity. The wrong guidance will make one's illness worse and may even bring about death. Therefore, look for a teacher who is well known in the medical community and who has tractable records for his teaching and guidance.

A teacher not only instructs a student through verbal communication and physical direction but through spiritual guidance as well. If the student is not honest with self and others, he or she will not be able to connect with the master. The student must also follow the direction of the teacher without doubt. Typically, ten months of instruction are required before one learns to increase the flow of energy in the body. However, a good teacher can double the rate in which the energy flows.

A good teacher also maximizes his students' comprehension of the diverse principles of Qigong, which combine such fields as philosophy, biology, psychology, geology, astrology, medicine, mathematics and music.

During the physical exercises, the more one focuses on the teacher the more one connects with the spiritual energy of the teacher. The energy becomes a force that opens the mind and simulates the brain. This stimulation of brain activity has been known to be so intense that people become able to heal physically or to perform physical deeds that appear miraculous. If one cannot achieve this state, the essence of Qigong cannot be comprehended.

For the student it is important to understand the gifts of knowledge and skill the teacher has given. Students will therefore want to return a favor ten fold to a teacher. If the mind, body and soul are open to the teacher and the student will accept the strict discipline of the teacher, he or she will absorb all that the teacher has to offer. An ancient Chinese proverb says that if one works truly hard an iron rod can be ground into a needle.

Respect must always be given to teachers and elders. Always be humble, conscientious, and forthright with others. Remember, when receiving a favor, always give back more than what was given to you.

ENLIGHTENMENT

The Chinese character for "enlightenment" is a combination of the symbols for five and door. Qigong allows you to

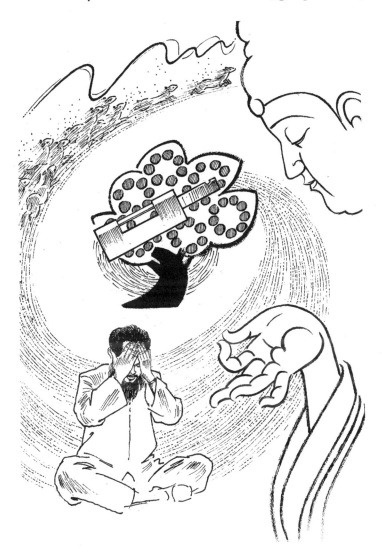

Unlocking -- inspirational meditation

achieve enlightenment of the body when the five doorways of the body (head, hands, and feet) open to receive or absorb energy and knowledge. The five doorways are integral to healing since they are also connected to the five major organs of the body.

This state of enlightenment is also integral to exercises such as tai chi, meditation, and martial arts. Enlightenment is indicated by numbness, tingling sensations, or sweat. These responses mean that energy is flowing throughout the body. Enlightenment allows for the channeling of energy and the building of a strong immune system, as well as increasing intellectual ability and improving endurance. When studying the theory of Qigong, do not go about it logically as a computer would, but try to internalize the teachings and try to understand its fundamental principles.

While many people who study Qigong are open and accepting, some have doubts and may even be resistant. Those that are resistant will obviously regain health at a slower rate.

Human beings are combinations of bio-energy systems, bio-magnetic fields, and bio-electrical waves. The bio-electrical wave can transfer thought from one human to another. For example, when a parent is dying, a child in a distant location may feel major physical and emotional reactions, sensing that something is wrong. A bio-wave connection has therefore been made. Similar principles can be found in the Qigong energy exercises. The relationship between the teacher and the student can parallel that of a walkie-talkie. When people are open to each other, clear communication is possible. Once this level of openness is achieved, enlightenment occurs and help is transferred.

WISDOM

Wisdom is often recognized under opposing circumstances. A person can suddenly achieve wisdom under pressure or in the last moment of life. Wisdom also comes when one is calm and the mind is at peace.

A person at the final moment of life may be awakened to the knowledge that the full potential of the mind can be accessed. Similarly, when the mind is calm, quiet and empty, the person can also access the mind's full potential. This theory can be seen in a famous Chinese novel, *Journey to the West*, in which the three main characters are "Enlightenment of Emptiness," "Enlightenment of Calm," and "Enlightenment of Power."

The Qigong practitioner will attain wisdom through calm and quiet. While practicing Qigong, some people see vague images while their eyes are closed. This experience suggests that one is tapping into the psychic abilities of the mind. Signs frequently foretell events. For example, before the onset of an earthquake birds will squeak, mice will run and lakes will bubble. Likewise, if the practitioner can sense the energy of the universe, he or she will be able to absorb the magnetic fields of heaven and earth for the enhancement of wisdom.

HELPING OTHERS

Charity and selflessness are central to Qigong. The sun and the earth constantly give forth energy and never ask for payment. Qigong teaches respect for parents combined with faith, passion, honesty, sincerity, love, kindness, fairness, consideration, mercy and peace. Righteousness starts with helping others. In today's society, many seek materialistic relationships and have materialistic goals. However, Qigong practitioners operate on the principle that giving is better than receiving and give to people who have asked for help without expecting repayment of any kind. By helping others one attains happiness that strengthens the ability to perform the Qigong exercises. When one helps others the universe provides help in return. Throughout the world and across time, this principle of doing good deeds holds true.

When practicing Qigong in today's society, the student should observe and understand the self before using Qigong skills. When reactions or sensations during exercise are not experienced, one should re-evaluate the practice in order to be sure it is correct. By being calm and patient in the practice of Qigong, the student should harvest benefits within two to three months.

PART TWO

GENERAL QIGONG
EXERCISES

There are six general Qigong exercise sets that I have designed for people with different needs. Students or patients should choose the most appropriate sets for their practice according to their own situations.

12

The Dragon Restoring Qi Exercises

This Qigong set can restore the Primary Qi (good, positive, and life sustaining Qi from the universe) of the body in a very short period of time, enabling the internal *yin-yang* balance of one's Qi and blood. It is most effective in treating the following conditions: diseases of the digestive system, kidney disease, neck and spinal problems, hair loss, bursitis, and various lung and heart diseases, such as bronchitis, expansion of bronchus, coughing, asthma, hemoptysis, coronary heart disease, pneumosilicosis, flu, etc.

BODY MOVEMENTS

1.   (Preparation) Stand with feet apart at shoulders' width. Visualize the feet extending into the core of the earth. Relax the whole body but do not hunch. Tuck in the hips, lift the anus and the kidneys. The hands hang naturally on both sides. The eyes look to the front. Visualize that the sky, the earth,

61

and the human body have become one. Recite (say aloud) the five sounds: *Ju-e—, Zh-i—, G-o-ng—, Sh-a-ng—, Y-u—*. With each sound, try to feel the vibration in the corresponding organ (i.e. liver, heart, spleen, lungs, and kidneys, respectively). Sub-vocalize (say silently) the five notes again three times, and feel any sensations in the organs. Bring each sound, together with the saliva, down to the lower abdomen (lower *Dantian* area).

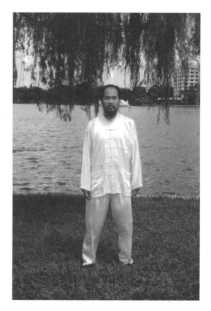

2.   Clasp your hands with the knuckles towards the earth and palms towards each other in front of the lower abdomen (the lower *Dantian*). Relax and feel the gathering and merging of the human body's internal Qi, and the sky and Earth's external Qi. Visualize the opening up of the following body points: the *Lao Gong* points (at the center of the palms), the *Yong Quan* points (at the center of the soles of the feet), and the *Bai Hui* point (at the top of the head).

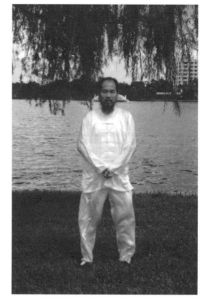

Inhale with the nose while gently lifting the hands up along the centerline of the front of the body (the *Ren* meridian) until the chest level is reached (the middle *Dantian*). Do not pause here.

3. From the chest level, rotate the clasped hands so that the knuckles are on top. Continue to bring the hands upwards. Follow them with your eyes and slightly tilt the head back as they move past the eye level. Also rotate the hands until the intertwined palms open up to face the sky and the arms are fully extended. At that point, stretch your body position vertically and hold for a couple of seconds. Visualize yourself standing on the earth and supporting the sky. Then look to the front and resume the head position.

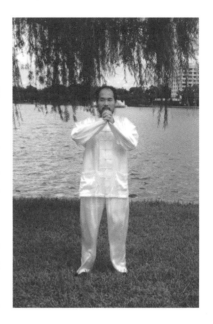

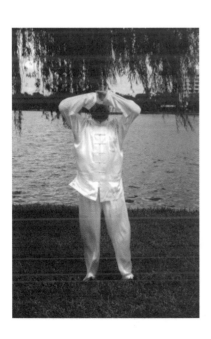

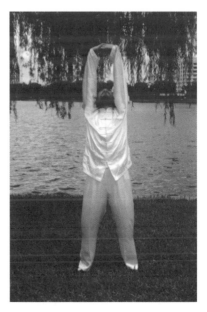

4. Separate the hands and bring them down gently on each side to the shoulder level, with the palms facing outward and the arms relaxed but still extended. Exhale through the nose during this movement. Stretch and hold that position for a couple of seconds.

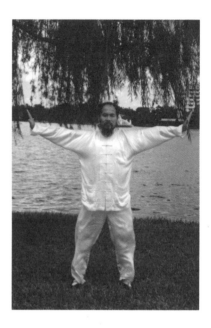

5. Slowly rotate the hands and arms so that the palms face the front and the fingers point outward. Bring the hands forward and then inward toward the lower abdomen, visualizing the gathering and drawing of the positive and good energy from the earth, sky, and human world into the lower *Dantian*. As the hands come toward the

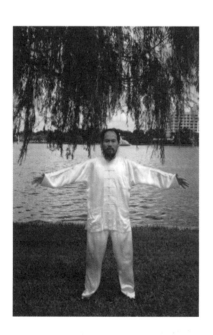
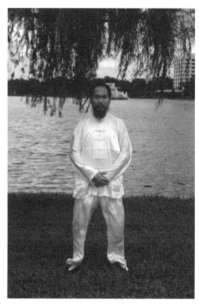

lower abdomen, the gentleman places his left hand on the lower *Dantian*, and his right palm on top of it. The lady places her right hand on the lower *Dantian*, and her left palm on top of it.

6.   Gently resume the clasped hand position and repeat Steps 2 to 5 for several times.

Closing Process after Each Exercise

7.   Remain relaxed with your eyes closed. Rub the palms of both hands until they become hot.

8.   Bring the palms to your chin and rub your face with an upward motion until you reach the hair line on your forehead while inhaling.

9.   Then bring your palms in a downward motion to the starting point while exhaling (similar to washing one's face). Complete this process nine times and on the last (the downward) process, continue rubbing from the chin down to just below the navel (*Dantian* area where all energy is stored).

10.   Place the right hand on the left hand and hold for a while in order to store the energy acquired during the exercise (for females the left hand must be placed on the right hand). Take a deep breath and holding it for a few moments while retaining the hands on the *Dantian* area. Complete this process three times. The process contributes toward smooth skin and

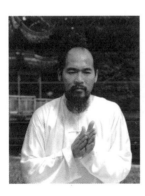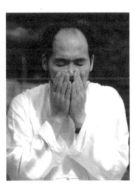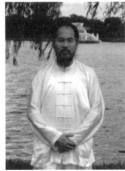

assists in elimination of wrinkles from the face. Inhale three times and swallow the saliva with the Qi down to the lower *Dantian* as you exhale through the nose.

Qi Movements

1. To begin, initiate the body's internal Qi movement. Open up the *Ren* meridian (along the centerline on the front of

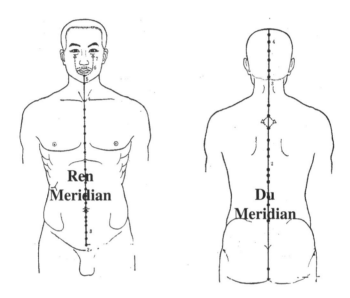

the body) and *Du* meridian (along the centerline on the back of the body). Open the body points: *Bai Hui* (at the top of the head), *Lao Gong* (at the center of each palm) and *Yong Quan* (at

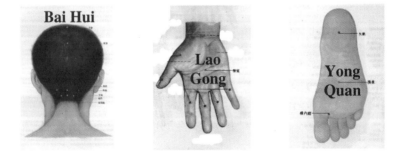

the center of each sole). Begin to receive and communicate in the Qi-level between the sky, the earth, and the human world.

2. The silent communication and transfer of sound and saliva to the lower *Dantian* (in the lower abdomen) generates warmth and heat. Qi and the five notes (corresponding to the five internal organs) produce energy that further promotes the movement of the body's Primary Qi. With both feet stepping willingly "into" the earth, the Qi circulates up and down the whole body and refreshes the system.

3. When the hands are placed at the lower *Dantian* at the start of the movement, the Primary Qi at the lower abdomen begins to gather and accumulate. Bringing the hands up subsequently moves the Primary Qi from the lower *Dantian* to the middle *Dantian* (the chest level) and to the upper *Dantian* (the level of the eyebrows).

4. Extending the hands above the head moves the Primary Qi from the shoulder level through the elbows, the forearms, the wrists, the *Lao Gong* points (at the center of each palm), and to the ten fingers. When the palms face the sky, the Primary Qi passes along the ten fingers and the hands are "holding up the sky," assuming the posture of "Standing on Earth and Supporting the Sky."

5. After that, the Primary Qi goes back to the *Lao Gong* points through the ten fingers. At this time, the *Lao Gong* points breathe as the Universe (sky, earth, and human world) does, exchanging energy to promote the body's metabolism.

6. When both arms are extended out to either side of the body, the body expels the bad and negative internal Qi through the three main body points (*Bai Hui*, *Lao Gong*, and *Yong Quan*). After the elimination of the bad Qi, the whole body feels good. Positive Qi dominates and circulates within the body. At this time, the *Lao Gong* points of each hand inhale and gather the positive and good Qi from nature and the universe into the body, passing through the head level (upper *Dantian*), the chest level (middle *Dantian*) and settling down deep into the lower abdomen (lower *Dantian*).

WORDS FROM THE MASTER

1. This Qigong set looks simple, however one should try to understand its meaning: To receive the *yang* energy from the sky, combine the Primary Qi from the human world, and receive the *yin* energy from the earth, so as to initiate and induce one's energy.

2. If one can master its meaning and also practice diligently, this Qigong set can open up doors to our various potentials, in addition to building up an excellent respiratory system. The same is true for the other Qigong sets that follow.

3. This Qigong set opens up body points and promotes the communication between the body-mind and the universe during the "bodily breathing." Inhale when bringing up the hands from the lower *Dantian*. Exhale when bringing the hands

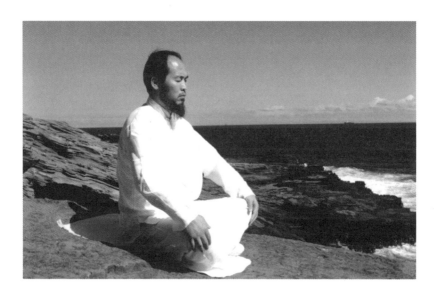

down on either side of the body. (Also exhale through the *Lao Gong* points on the palms, expelling the negative and bad Qi from within). Inhale again when bringing the hands forward and then inward toward the abdomen, gathering the good and positive Qi from the sky, the earth, and the human world to supplement the body's lost energy. When the hands are covering the lower abdomen, exhale and return the Qi back to the lower *Dantian*. For beginners, this Qigong set can treat illnesses and promote health. As one reaches an advanced stage, this Qigong set enables the development of extraordinary potentials and promotes communication between everything in the universe.

FEELINGS AND RESULTS

1. One may feel a hot sensation along the back, the abdomen, the palms, the fingers, and even around the whole body. One may also feel a sensation of numbness and swelling on the palms.

2. One may feel a twitching and warming sensation on the feet, the hands, the face, and the lower abdomen.

3. After practicing for a period of time, the *Ren* and *Du* meridians (along the centerline on the front and back of the body) open up and Qi flows freely. One may feel that his or her spirit becomes very positive, limitless, and alive, matching that of the sky and the earth.

13

The Phoenix and the Rising Sun Exercises

This Qigong set effectively treats joint pain, leg and foot pain, diseases related to the urinary system, hemorrhoids, prolapse of anus, etc. It also strengthens the kidneys and treats gynecological problems.

BODY MOVEMENTS

1. Preparation: Stand with feet apart at shoulder width. Visualize the feet extending into the core of the earth. Relax the whole body but do not hunch. Tuck in the hips, lift the anus and (visually) the kidneys. Hands hang naturally on both sides. Eyes look to the front. Visualize that the sky, the earth, and the human body have become one. Recite (say aloud) the five sounds: *Ju-e—, Zh-i—, G-o-ng—, Sh-a-ng—, Y-u—*. With each sound, try to feel the vibration in the corresponding organ (i.e. liver, heart, spleen, lungs, and kidneys). Sub-vocalize (say silently) the five sounds again for three times and feel the organs. Bring each sound, together with the saliva, down to the lower

abdomen (lower *Dantian* area).

2. Spread the legs to assume a wider stance and bend
the knees slightly. Visualize the
feet extending into the core of
the earth. Straighten the back
but do not expose the chest.
Eyes look to the front. Both
arms extend horizontally to the
front. The palms face forward
and the fingers are vertical just
like the phoenix fanning up her
feathers.

3. Closing: Rub your

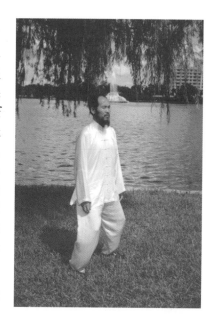

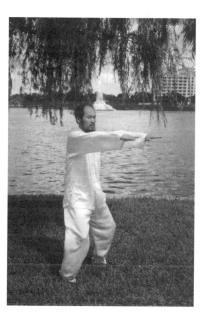
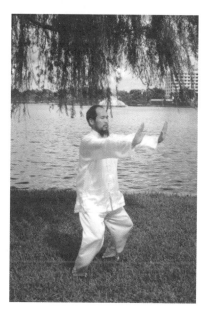

palms together until hot, then "wash" your face with the Qi on
your palms. Massage your ears and pat your head. Inhale three

times, recite the five sounds (with the mouth shut), and swallow the saliva with the Qi (and the sound) down to the lower *Dantian* as you exhale through the nose.

Qi Movements

1.   During this Qigong set, use subtle strength with the thighs and the calves so that the Primary Qi circulates without constriction. Relax the whole body so the Primary Qi can circulate throughout the body.

2.   This Qigong set enables the movement of internal Qi, opens the twelve main meridians (energy channels), and opens the eight extra-meridians.

Words from the Master

1.   This Qigong exercise looks like a quiescent type Qigong with a bent-knee stance. However, it has the essence of those quiescent-external and dynamic-internal Qigong types. It restores the balance of the body's internal *yin-yang*. This apparently simplistic Qigong movement demands the practitioners' concentration and dedication in order to absorb the positive energy from the sky and the earth.

2.   During inhalation, visualize the absorption of all forms of energy (light, heat, electricity, magnetism, sound, waves, etc.) from the sun through the *Lao Gong* points (center of the palms), along the arms and into the lower *Dantian* of the body. Because of the ample emission of solar energy from 5-7 a.m. in the morning, facing and gathering energy from the sun at dawn yields the best result. During exhalation, visualize the release of bad and negative Qi from top to bottom via the meridians of the whole body passing through legs and feet, and out into the ground through the *Yong Quan* points (center of the sole of the feet).

3.   The breathing method for this Qigong set is the Re-

verse Abdominal breathing style. When inhaling, lift the anus and (visually) the kidneys, and contract the lower abdomen. Visualize the absorption of all kinds of positive energy from the Sun and the universe into the body, through the *Lao Gong* points (and all other body points) into the lower *Dantian*. When exhaling, relax the lower abdomen.

4.　　The eyes look forward as if gazing in spirit at the universe. Feel the positive Qi of the body. Visualize breathing through the pores all over the body. Breathe the Primary Qi (good, positive, and life sustaining Qi from the universe) into the body and channel it along the invisible line through the three *chakras* (the three bodily or spiritual centers: the top of the head, the chest area, and the perineum). Feel the abundance of the positive Qi, within and without the human body, achieving the grand state of "Qi within Body and Body within Qi." Feel the organs inside the body being fueled with energy one after another, causing a holistic readjustment of the human body. At this point, the body is one with the universe.

5.　　The mind is cleansed and selfless, the look of the eyes

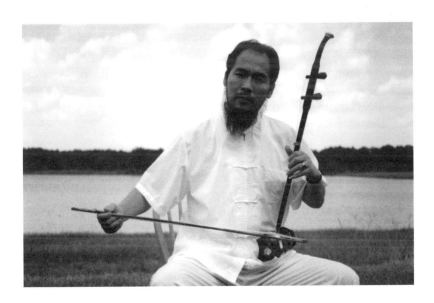

commanding of awe. The body is strong as a foundation rock and sturdy as Mount Tai (a very famous high mountain in China). Successful practitioners of this Qigong set will have their Qigong strength increased, their bone marrow growth improved, and their body and mind harmonized.

FEELINGS AND RESULTS

1. This Qigong set promotes Qi circulation along the meridians of the whole body, adjusting and harmonizing excess and deficiency in the human body, including over-weight and under-weight conditions.

2. This Qigong set clears up the meridians between the heart, the liver, and the gallbladder. It also promotes audacity, which, according to Chinese medicine, has something to do with the gallbladder.

3. It rids the body of negative energy and supplements it with positive energy. It also changes the persona and personal qualities of a person while improving patience, manner of thinking, and level of creativity.

4. It cleanses the mind and the heart, healing emotional problems.

14

Converging
Energy Exercises

This Qigong set effectively treats insomnia, hypertension, arrhythmia (irregular heartbeat), and other diseases of the nervous system. It also treats tumors resulting from diseases of the liver, gallbladder, digestive system, and stomach, as well as heart diseases, diabetes, and cancer.

BODY MOVEMENTS

The exercises in this set can be done while standing, sitting, or lying down on the back.

1. Relax the whole body. Calm down the mind. Have the eyes almost closed. Wear a smile on the face. Visualize and recite silently for three times the five sounds: *Ju-e—*, *Zh-i—*, *G-o-ng—*, *Sh-a-ng—*, *Y-u—*. Sink the sound with the breath and saliva into the lower *Dantian* (lower abdomen area).

2. Place both hands close together, but not touching each other, in front of the abdomen. Have the fingers close to, but not touching, one another on each hand and start to pull the hands apart slowly and evenly. Each finger should be relaxed. The movement is like pulling a rubber band on both sides, but with the fingers not touching one another. At the same time, have the toes on both feet curl toward the ground, as if grabbing the earth. It is best to do this while listening to the Qigong music.

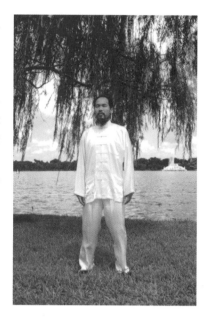

3. When both hands are apart the farthest distance possible without tensing up the movement, open up the palm and start drawing the hands and palms toward each other, again slowly and evenly. Each finger

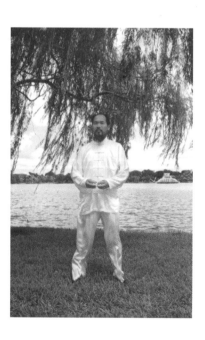

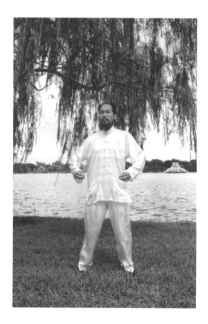

should be relaxed. This movement is like compressing a
spring. At the same time, relax
the toes. When the hands almost touch each other in front
of the abdomen, repeat Step 2.

4. Use natural breathing
for this Qigong set. Exhale
while the hands draw away
from each other and inhale
while they come toward each
other. One exhalation and one
inhalation complete one movement cycle.

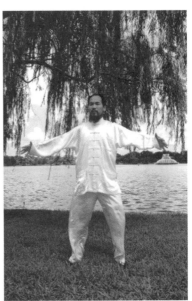

5. Closing: When done,
return both hands to the lower abdomen. Consolidate and return the energy to the lower *Dantian*. Rub your palms together
until hot, then "wash" your face with the Qi on your palms.
Massage your ears and pat your
head. Inhale three times, recite
the five sounds (with the mouth
shut), and swallow the saliva
with the Qi (and the sound)
down to the lower *Dantian* as
you exhale through the nose.

Qi Movements

1. The ten fingers draw
apart and together as softly as
handling silk. All finger joints
should be relaxed. The whole
hand movement should look
fluid, smooth, and natural.

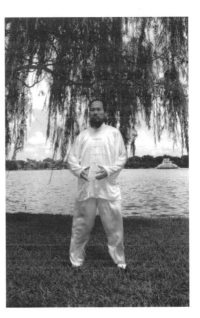

2. The ten toes clench the ground when the fingers are close to one another. They relax when the palms open up.

3. This Qigong set harmonizes and facilitates the Qi flow along the twelve main meridians of the body: three hand *yin* meridians, three hand *yang* meridians, three foot *yin* meridians, and three foot *yang* meridians. It opens up the meridians and enhances their functions.

WORDS FROM THE MASTER

1. The ten fingers and the ten toes are the beginning points or the end points of the twelve main meridians. They are connected to the eight extra meridians, and have a direct connection to the five *yin* organs and the six *yang* organs. The five *yin* organs are the liver, the heart, the spleen, the lungs, and the kidneys. The six *yang* organs are the gallbladder, the small intestine, the stomach, the large intestine, the urinary bladder, and the pericardium.

2. The ten fingers and the ten toes directly gather and absorb the Primary Qi from the sky and the earth into the *yin*

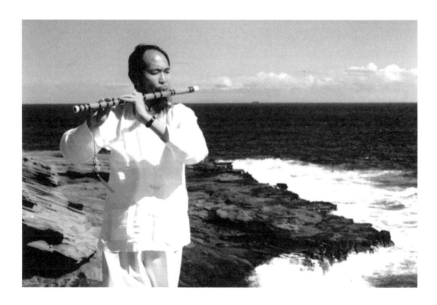

and *yang* internal organs of the body. The movement harmonizes and facilitates the Qi flow along the meridians and can strengthen the constitution of the practitioner. When the ten fingers (and toes) draw together while the hands pull apart, Primary Qi from the universe is gathered and stored in the lower *Dantian*. When the palms open up and toes relaxed, Qi circulates normally along the twelve meridians. This Qigong set can augment greatly the quality of one's Qi base and can build up one's foundation for higher level Qigong practices.

FEELINGS AND RESULTS

1. This Qigong set allows the practitioner to feel the Qi quickly and strongly. It opens up the cerebral functions and cultivates intelligence. It also promotes the coordination between the brain and the four limbs.

2. It increases the power of the ten fingers and the ten toes.

3. Possible results include a feverish and swelling sensation over the whole body, a twitching sensation in the coccyx and perineum area, internal vision (i.e. one can see inward toward one's skeletal structure or internal organs), the feeling of a shining bead rolling inside the lower *Dantian*, etc. Through the coordination of the ten fingers and the ten toes during the Qigong practice, the *yin-yang* harmony of internal organs can be harmonized. This Qigong set enhances the digestive system and promotes the blood and Qi circulation and transformation through the body.

15

The Receptive Soul Exercises

Mental Preparation: First, free your mind from any limiting thoughts. Abandon your usual way of cognitive and logical thinking. Discard any selfishness. Empty your mind so that it is like a blank cassette tape. It is like a balloon with a vacuum in it, truly staying in a state of ultimate silence and all-dimensional soul reception.

Enter this space in our universe where matters are immaterial energy. They are spiritual and weightless. They are not affected by the Earth's gravity. If we humans successfully communicate with this spiritual matrix, we can then arrive at a state of peaceful void. We will be able to use our spiritual agility, our spiritual heart, and our spiritual sincerity to sense and receive the truth of Musical Qigong. And we will discover new things in our world.

PHYSICAL POSTURE

Assume the cross-legged sitting position, or sit on a chair

with the legs naturally touching the ground. Place both palms towards each other (Imagine you hold the earth, male left palm on top, female right palm on top).

To avoid external distractions, keep your mind peaceful. Have your eyes almost closed, and relax. Relax each and every part of your body one after the other. First, relax your head, eyes, nose, mouth, ears, every part of it. Then relax as follows: neck, shoulders, internal organs, hips, thighs, knees, calves and feet. Also relax all major pressure points (or acupuncture points) located along the *Ren* and *Du* meridians (the centerline on the front and back of the body) from top to bottom. Alternatively, if you don't know their locations, you can just relax three times from top to bottom your body centerline in front, and three times from top to bottom the centerline on your back. Afterwards, relax all meridians of your body.

When you are familiar with the above relaxation techniques, you will be able to relax each and every piece of your body's flesh and bone. At this time, slowly visualize a quiet relaxed state of void within your body. Feel that the sky and earth are peaceful and quiet, that the universe is also peaceful and quiet, all in a state of void.

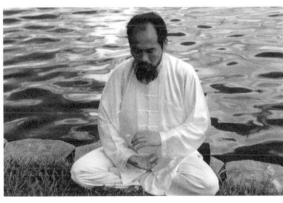

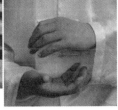

BREATHING

Many people erroneously believe that the physical act of breathing is done by the lungs. Actually, the lungs cannot expand and contract on their own. The act of breathing relies on the diaphragm and the intercostal muscles. When the muscles expand the thoracic cavity, air is forced into the lungs through the trachea and bronchi by atmospheric pressure. Similarly, when the muscles cause a reduction in the size of the thoracic cavity, air is forced out of the lungs.

Now, adjust your breathing according to these mechanics. During inhalation, naturally breathe in the air (Qi) through the nose into the body. During exhalation, visualize sinking the Qi down to the lower abdomen. Make your breathing slow, small, long and even. If you master these techniques, you will benefit from this Qigong set immediately.

THE FIVE-NOTE INCANTATION

If the incantation one chooses is true and realistic, representative of his or her wish and belief, and capable of promoting his or her success, then he or she will non-defensively and pleasantly accept and internalize the incantation. Therefore, recite the five-note incantation silently when you enter Qigong state during your practice of the Receptive Soul Qigong set. When your mind is focused and your cognition is pure, silently recite the incantation that can produce strong power toward achieving your goals. Concentrate and chisel into your clear mind the substantial question that awaits resolution. Recite silently the five sounds: *Gong, Shang, Jue, Zhi, Yu*. At the same time, focus your mind on the corresponding organ. Feel your spleen during the *Gong* sound. Feel your lungs during the *Shang* sound. Feel your liver during the *Jue* sound. Feel your heart during the *Zhi* sound, and feel your kidneys during the *Yu* sound. Do not recite aloud. Recite deep within your heart slowly and silently, again and again. Use subsonic waves to act on your internal organs and cause harmonic resonance, promoting the body's immune system. The incantation, also called True Words, has mystical power. Following the five notes and entering into this ultimate serene state will allow oneself to be more receptive of any external messages within a very short time, resulting in a merged unity of oneself and the mystical power.

Note One: When treating children with a wide variety of diseases, please play the Qigong music while the children are sleeping. This will yield exceptional results because when children are asleep, their meridians and points are relaxed and more susceptible to receiving sonic energy and Qigong messages.

Note Two: For bed-ridden patients and those who cannot take care of themselves, listening to Qigong music while practicing the Receptive Soul Qigong set constitutes a very effective treatment. It promotes restoration of the cerebral cortex, massages the internal organs, clears up meridians, and regulates Qi and blood within the body.

Gong   **Shang**   **Jue**   **Zhi**   **Yu**

宫　　　商　　　角　　　徵　　　羽

16

The Sleeping Wiseman Exercises

This is a particularly effective exercise for those who are being confined to bed due to movement limitation; or it can be a quick and easy way for anyone to receive and revitalize his or her energy. I also call it the lazy man's answer to Qigong for its low effort nature. When performed correctly, one can practice and receive energy just by lying down. Since the exercise is simplistic in nature, I offer only a brief description.

BODY MOVEMENTS

There are two ways to do this exercise, and they are equally effective. You can either lie on your side (top, next page), or on your back (bottom, next page). If you choose to lie on your side, I encourage you to lie on your right side so as to avoid putting any pressure on your heart, especially those who have any heart related conditions. For those who suffer from any liver related condition, I advise that you lie on your back.

84

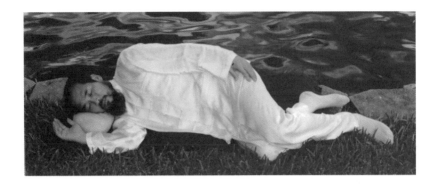

Following the basic requirements from the previous exercises (proper breathing, emptying mind, etc.), lie on your right side in a relaxed and natural position with your chin slightly in and your right arm bent at a 90 degree position next to your face. The head is supported comfortably with a pillow. Your right palm should be opened facing the sky with your thumb and your index finger connecting at the tips forming a circle. Legs are slightly bent with the left leg on top of the right leg. Your left arm should be lying naturally and comfortably on your left hip with palm facing downward.

QI MOVEMENTS

With the Qigong music playing, breathe comfortably and naturally through your nose. Imagine that you are breathing in all the energy from above through the eye (center point) of

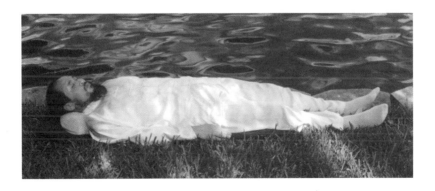

your right palm and through the pores on your skin. Visualize that you are absorbing all the energy from the music into your body like a baby receiving nourishment in the mother's womb. Let the energy slowly drift down to your lower abdomen, or *Dantian*, and store it there.

To practice this exercise on your back requires virtually the same technique, except that one should lie on his or her back with arms lying naturally and comfortably on the sides, palms facing down.

WORDS FROM THE MASTER

Avoid over eating or hunger during practice, for either condition may affect your concentration.

The air in the room should be well circulated, but avoid strong, direct breeze. Maintain proper room temperature and comfortable lighting.

17

Guan-yin Aided Natural Adjustment Exercises

The main function of this Qigong set is to discard our "shallow" consciousness and dig into our "deeper" consciousness.

Most people know Guan-yin as the Goddess of Mercy. In Chinese, the words "Guan" and "Yin" also mean "observe" and "sound or music" respectively. As its name implies, this Qigong aims at allowing the music to induce the vigor of *yang* Qi within the body, eventually causing different parts of the body to move and dance spontaneously. This is a type of natural movement spontaneity dance. Although this Qigong movement is spontaneous, it is not haphazard; it promotes the opening of energy channels.

First, stand naturally while listening to the medicinal meditation Qigong music. Get prepared for doing the Guan-yin Aided Natural Adjustment Qigong set.

Allow yourself to experience the effect on you by the sur-

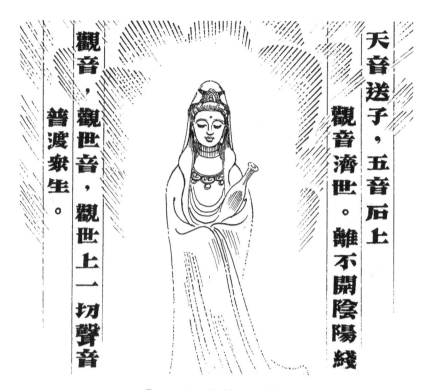

天音送子，五音后上
觀音濟世。離不開陰陽綫

觀音，觀世音，觀世上一切聲音
普渡衆生。

Guanyin, Goddess of Mercy

rounding light, electricity, magnetism, waves, and sound. Understand that you also have an effect upon these surrounding energies. Allow yourself to merge with heaven (sky), earth, and man, sharing the same Qi. Unite with all under the universe, matching, complementing, and communicating with each other. Feel the mutual attractive force between nature and you.

When you hear the music, start by "sinking" your concentration to your lower *Dantian* (abdomen). At the same time, "observe" the sound – a biorhythmic vibration – from your lower *Dantian*. Relax your whole body and observe the sound, "Guan-yin." Recite silently the words "Guan-yin … Guan-yin …" while keeping a calm and even breathing.

At the beginning, you may feel your body rocking back and

forth – from slight to more substantial movement, from a localized area to the whole body, from vigorous intensity to a more balanced state, from moving haphazardly to rhythmically, from movements with occasional pauses to those with voluntary pauses and re-starts. Do not get nervous. Follow the method below and you will eventually realize the internal truth and value of this Qigong set.

When your body starts rocking back and forth, do not apply "mental energy" to control it. At this time, your body may start to produce movements of different styles similar to martial arts, kung fu, tai chi, operatic moves, or dance steps. You may spontaneously pat, hit, nudge, massage, or poke at yourself. You may do exercise, dance, or make noise. Each person will do something according to his or her body's needs and no two "dance steps" are completely the same. Movement of the body and limbs follows a normal pattern: observe the sound – serenity – spontaneous external movement – external movement pauses while internal movement keeps going – the state of the big void (emptiness).

When your movement stops, you will feel a very pleasant sensation, and a great ease into meditation. At this time, you should quickly focus your mind on your lower *Dantian* (abdomen below the navel) to cause the Qi of the whole body to stay tightly at that location. Primary Qi goes in, and bad Qi comes out. Several minutes later, the rocking movement may reappear. Again keep the Qi to stay tightly at your *Dantian*.

If, after ten or more days of practice, you still do not feel any movements, it means that you are still not merged with the energy of this nature and universe. Be patient and keep practicing in a relaxed state.

This Qigong exercise should be used in combination with Shen Wu Medicinal Qigong music. The practice will move in a gradual progression toward communicating with nature, observing sound, light, and music, which in turn promotes the body's defense system.

Guan-yin Aided Natural Adjustment Qigong combines both quiescent and dynamic Qigong exercises. It enables a quick enhancement of our "Qi reservoir" and riddance of ailments. Because of the exchange of energy with the universe in terms of sound, light, electricity, heat, wave, magnetism, etc., this Qigong involves different types of Primary Qi and a natural medium of conduction and absorption. As a result, the mind and body energy of the practitioner is naturally adjusted.

In addition, while practicing this Qigong, the practitioner also experiences significant enjoyment. It is easier than other Qigong sets which require the practitioner to finish a certain number of particular movements within a given time.

When students are being taught face to face, it is not necessary to teach them the Qigong movements. The goal is to let them feel the Primary Qi by themselves. There are practitioners who have been practicing for years or even tens of years but still do not know what Qi really is or what it feels like, and their ailments have not improved. My Musical Qigong aims at allowing students to feel and realize what Qi is about within their own bodies, and to learn how to achieve special Qi manipulating techniques. Everything is done in a state of void (emptiness), naturally and without force or willful intent. Eventually the practitioner will be able to accomplish the following: know how to observe Qi, observe halo, see through substances, sense from a distance, treat illnesses from a distance, etc. These skills will occur naturally and without effort. They will allow one to release physical ailments and bad Qi while cultivating confidence in Qigong.

Qigong is a joyful practice.

PART THREE

QIGONG
EXERCISES FOR
THE FIVE ORGANS

These exercises contribute towards smooth skin and assist in elimination of wrinkles from the face.

PREPARATION

■　　Wear loose comfortable clothing, preferably made of silk. You can wear normal cloths but should remove anything that restricts blood flow such as tight belts, watches, shoes, etc.

■　　Prior to exercising, do not have a heavy meal or perform strenuous work, physical activities, etc.

■　　Do not exercise if you are angry. You will not be able to focus or concentrate on the exercises for anger will cause Qi energy flow disorder.

■　　Keep pets away while exercising as they may disturb you while you are in deep concentration. The sudden interruption or fright could cause damage to your kidneys.

■　　Schedule your exercises between 5 a.m. and 7 a.m. daily. This is the time when Qi energy is at its optimum, and it is also the time when your mind will be refreshed and concentration is a lot easier.

■　　Have Musical Qigong Therapeutical Collections (5 audio tapes) ready to be played appropriately for each exercise.

Note: Exercise Six does not require any music.

EXERCISES

☐   Sit on the front one third of the seat of a chair and rock from side to side and front to back until you find the most comfortable position.

☐   Spread your feet apart the same distance as the width between your shoulders. The knee joint should form a 90-degree angle as much as possible. The back should be straight with the shoulder relaxed.

☐   The exercises may also be performed while sitting on the floor with crossed legs and a straight back, or while standing. The tip of your tongue should slightly touch the roof of the mouth at the most forward point. The eyes must always be kept slightly closed during the exercises so as to improve concentration and to retain the acquired energy. Inhale and exhale through the nose.

CLOSING PROCESS AFTER EACH EXERCISE:

♦   Remain relaxed with your eyes closed. Rub the palms of both hands together until they become hot. Bring the palms to your chin and rub your face with an upward motion until you reach the hair line on your forehead while inhaling. Then bring your palms in a downward motion to the starting point while exhaling (similar to washing one's face).

♦   Perform these steps nine times and on the last (the downward) step, continue rubbing from the chin down to just below the navel (*Dantian* area, where all energy is stored). Place the right hand on the left hand and hold for a while in order to store the energy acquired during the exercise (for females the left hand must be placed on the right hand). Take a deep breath and hold it for a few moments while retaining the hands on the *Dantian* area.

♦   Perform these steps three times.

18

Exercise One:
For the Liver

Benefits: Improve and produce more blood. Beneficial for the liver and gallbladder meridians. Reduce or eliminate diseases associated with blood, high or low blood pressure, and heart diseases. Improve symptoms associated with headaches, insomnia, EB virus, mental health, Parkinson disease, and eye diseases. Also good for the pulse.

Location: Upper right side of abdomen

Musical Tone: Wood

METHOD:

After assuming the right position, try relaxing and focus your thoughts on the liver within your body. It is very important that you maintain such concentration in order to obtain the benefits of this exercise.

Then place both hands on your knees with the palms facing

down and the tips of your index finger aligned with the top of your kneecaps (Note: the fingers must be kept together and the thumbs must be allowed to fall naturally). The thumbs will automatically land on an acupressure point connected to the liver.

The objective is to massage this area with a circular motion by moving the entire hand in a smooth rotation around both knees ensuring that the acupressure points are massaged with the center of the palm of each hand.

Inhale through your nose slowly and constantly during the entire circular motion of the massage until you return to the starting point, then, exhale slowly while completing a second revolution in the same direction. This will constitute one complete revolution.

You have to complete 36 of these complete revolutions in the same direction (clockwise or counter-clockwise) and then perform another 36 complete revolutions in the opposite direction to complete this exercise. Then, complete the Closing Process as stated above.

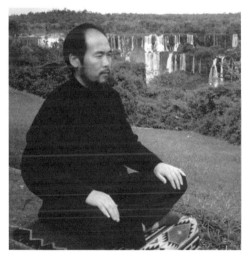
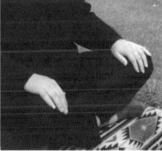

19

Exercise Two:
For the Heart

Benefits: Beneficial for the heart and small intestine meridians. Reduce or eliminate diseases associated with the heart, coronary diseases, high or low cholesterol, thick blood, heart blockage, stroke, irregular heartbeat, anxiety, stress, lack of concentration, secretion of small intestine, counteract negative energy, diseases of the spleen and stomach. In addition, it also calms overactive or scared kids, balances emotion, mind and energy.

Location: Chest cavity left of breastbone

Musical Tone: Fire

METHOD:

1.   After assuming the right position, try relaxing and fo-

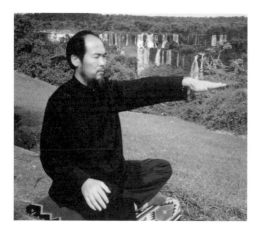

cus your thoughts on your heart within your body. Men should hold out their left hand in front of them at shoulder level with palms facing down. Women should hold out their right hand in a similar manner.

2. Rub the palm of the right hand lightly and slowly over the left arm, starting at the left shoulder and all the way down. The rubbing process will stimulate various meridians to accept energy. You must also inhale slowly and simultaneously turn your head to the right forming a 90-degree angle with your left arm.

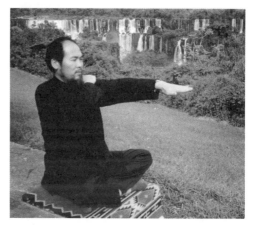

3. When your right palm reaches the tips of your left fingers, continue rubbing the underside of the left hand all the way up to the armpit while exhal-

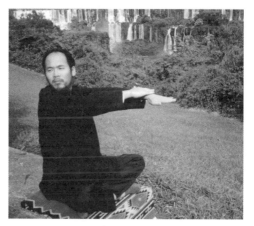

ing slowly. Also, slowly turn your head back to face forward.

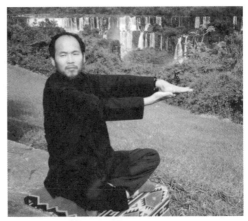

4. Bring the right palm to the heart area and apply some pressure momentarily, then, continue downward to your waist while still exhaling. This completes one cycle.

You must complete 36 of these cycles and then complete another 36 cycles using the opposite hand.

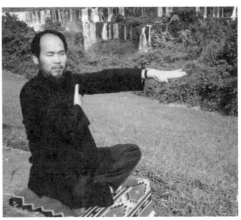

Then, complete the Closing Process as stated above.

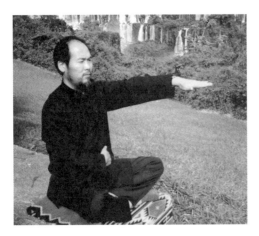

Note: Should you experience fatigue while holding out your hand, you may break up the exercise in smaller segments while changing hands until the 36 cycles are completed for each hand.

20

Exercise Three: For the Spleen

Benefits: Beneficial for the spleen and stomach meridians. Reduce or eliminate diseases associated with the digestive track, spleen and stomach. Improve symptoms associated with ulcers, upset stomach, heartburn, gas, burping, poison in the intestine, teeth problems, headaches, nutrients not being absorbed.

Location: Upper left side of abdomen

Musical Tone: Earth

METHOD:

After assuming the right position, try relaxing and focus your thoughts on your spleen within your body.

For men, place the palm of the left hand on the stomach area

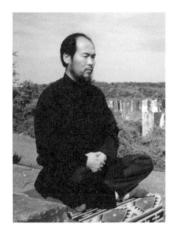

(just above the navel) and the palm of the right hand on the left hand. Women must do the opposite by placing the right hand first and the left hand on the right hand.

At this point both hands should be rubbed lightly and slowly in a circular motion (clockwise or counterclockwise) around the navel while inhaling slowly until you reach the starting point.

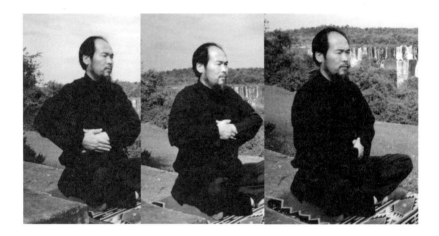

Continue another revolution in the same direction while exhaling slowly until you reach the starting point again.

This will constitute two revolutions, however, you must complete 36 revolutions in one direction (clockwise, or counterclockwise) and another 36 revolutions in the opposite direction. Then, complete the Closing Process as stated above.

100

21

Exercise Four:
For the Lungs

Benefits: Beneficial for the lungs and large intestine meridians. Reduce or eliminate problems associated with bronchitis, pneumonia, asthma, intestinal bacteria, and toothache.

Location: Upper chest area

Musical Tone: Metal

METHOD:

After assuming the right position, try relaxing and focus your thoughts on the lungs within your body.

Place your hands on your knees with the palms facing upward. While taking a deep slow breath, simultaneously start:

- forming a tight fist with both hands;

- curling the toes of both feet inward as though grabbing the floor;

- trying pulling up your diaphragm towards your chest, and;

- contracting or tightening all muscles in your buttocks. Hold this position for a few moments then slowly start exhaling and releasing the

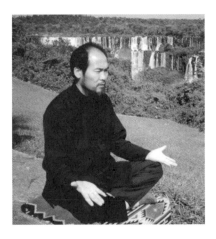

fists, toes (which should then be raised up), the organs and buttocks muscles.

This exercise should be completed the same number of times as your age multiplied by two.

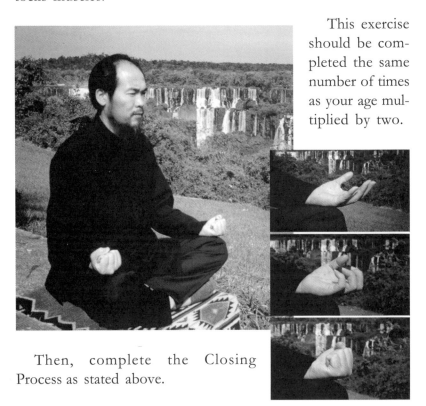

Then, complete the Closing Process as stated above.

22

Exercise Five:
For the Kidneys

Benefits: Beneficial for the kidney and urinary bladder meridians. Reduce or eliminate diseases associated with the uterus, prostate gland, urinary diseases, kidney stones, and diseases associated with the production organs.

Location: Half way down the back

Musical Tone: Water

METHOD:

After assuming the right position, try relaxing and focus on the kidneys within your body.

Bend forward and place the palms of both hands on your back at the highest point possible (top picture, next page).

While inhaling, slowly apply some pressure and slowly mas-

103

sage your back downward until you reach your buttocks (bottom picture).

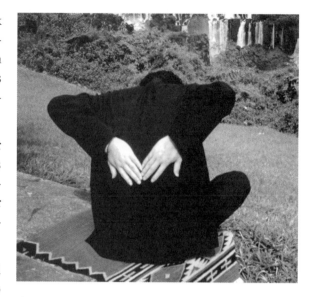

Hold your breath at this point and perform another cycle while exhaling slowly.

This will constitute two cycles and a total of 36 cycles are to be completed.

Then, complete the Closing Process as stated above.

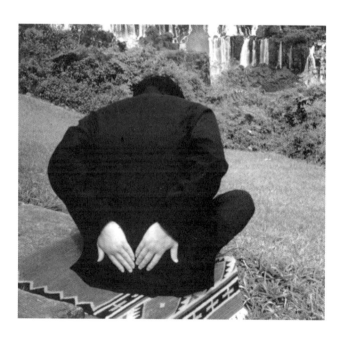

23

Exercise Six:
Expelling Bad Qi

These exercises should be done on a daily basis while playing the music of the five audio tapes. You should be feeling energized, rejuvenated and totally relaxed.

METHOD:

Stand with legs slightly bent, and fold fingers inward to form a small circle with the thumb and the forefinger of each hand.

Place the circle of the left hand on the stomach area and the circle of the right hand on your back directly opposite the left hand (this position is for males whereas females should use the opposite hands).

Strike the two areas simultaneously with a sharp blow (not to hurt yourself) while expelling all air from deep within your abdomen while saying "ha" loudly. This should be done several times while alternating hands.

Then, complete the Closing Process as stated above.

PART FOUR

LIFE MUSIC
FOR HEALING

Now let us get back to the concept of "five notes corresponding to the five internal organs" as mentioned in the first chapter. For the ancient Chinese people, the number "five" has a special meaning, and is incorporated into their culture, medicine, and philosophy. For daily life, they adopted a five-day cycle. For medicine, they correlated the five fingers on each hand to one of their five major internal organs, categorizing each organ according to the five elements—metal, wood, water, fire and earth.

It was according to the five elements theory of Chinese medicine that I have developed this five-piece Musical Qigong CD set. To achieve the best healing effect, the CDs should be listened to according to the following order:

♥   Monday: Shining Spring

♥   Tuesday: Receptive Souls

♥   Wednesday: A Journey in Harmony I

♥   Thursday: Heavenly Tunes

♥   Friday: A Journey in Harmony II

24

Shining Spring

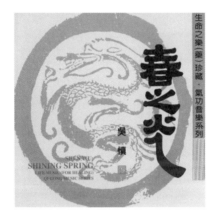

Monday—Jue—Wood—Liver

The springtime sunshine showers upon Mother Earth
and her people, bringing infinite hope and life.

The sound of the bamboo flute, a *Jue* (Wood) sound, is prominent on this CD. According to Chinese medicine, the wood sound opens and enters the energy channels of the liver and gallbladder of the human body, strengthening and enhancing them. Listening to these sounds can improve conditions related to anxiety, insomnia, night fright, failing memory, pallor, excessive thirst, vomiting, diarrhea, cold limbs, anemia, hepatitis, cirrhosis and other liver problems, inflammation of the gallbladder, gall stones, and other gallbladder problems. Women can experience reduction in pain related to conditions of the back and genitourinary tract. Additionally, "fetal education" in pregnant women is facilitated.

25

Receptive Souls

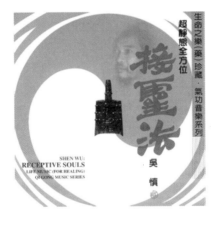

Tuesday—Zhi—Fire—Heart

This music incorporates the *Zhi* (Fire) sound which, ac
cording to Chinese medicine, opens and enters the energy channels of the heart and small intestine of the human

body. Listening to this music can relieve conditions such as chest stiffness, asthma with phlegm, eye fatigue, poor appetite, shoulder pain, wrist pain and numbness, heart problem, high and low blood pressure, palpitation, endocarditis, irregular heartbeat, enlarged heart muscles and other heart problems. It also has a beneficial effect on mental illnesses and pervasive insomnia. The opening of the heart has also been found to enhance one's physical beauty.

26

A Journey in Harmony I

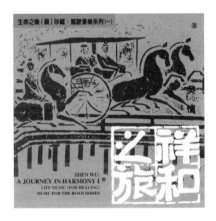

Wednesday—Gong—Earth—Spleen

This CD adopts the various melodies and rhythms of the central province of China along the Yellow River, where the ancient Chinese civilization originated. Their music was composed mainly of the *Gong* sound.

Gong music corresponds to the earth element. According to Chinese medicine, the *Gong* sound opens and enters the energy channels of the spleen and stomach of the human body, improving their overall functioning. The following conditions can be improved: poor appetite, anxiety, nausea, cold limbs, numbness, problems of the autonomic nervous system, stomach ulcers, chronic enteritis and other digestive disorders, constipation, deficiency of platelets in plasma, and dizziness. *Gong* music also supplements Qi and blood.

27

Heavenly Tunes

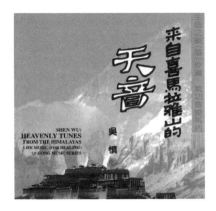

Thursday—Shang—Metal—Lungs

Hig「igh in the Himalayas, energy is received along the short-est path from the sun to the earth. This makes the sun's energy at that point the strongest. The pristine air and environment of the Himalayas is the cleanest, clearest, and pur-

115

est found on earth. The pure ice melting at the summit of the Himalayan mountain range creates the source for great rivers below that extend to many faraway lands. It is this strongest, purest, and most powerfully creative energy that the composer has transformed into music for the listener's enjoyment. The invigorating and uplifting energy of this music is sure to enhance the health, energy, and overall well-being of the listener.

The music of the piano, a stringed instrument prominently featured on this CD, correlates with the metal element.

According to Chinese medicine, the *Shang* (Metal) sound opens and enters the energy channels of the lungs and large intestine of the human body. Metal sounds can be used to improve the following conditions: palpitations, wrist numbness, the common cold, shoulder pain, sore throat, diarrhea, nerve pain of the wrist and face, nausea, vomiting, pulmonary emphysema, asthma, pneumonia, pulmonary tuberculosis and other lung problems, night sweats, toothaches, headaches, and dysentery.

28

A Journey in Harmony II

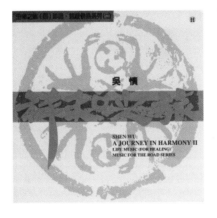

Friday—Yu—Water—Kidneys

The strong, powerful sound of the drum is heard in this CD. The music corresponds to the water element.

In Chinese medical tradition, the *Yu* (Water) sound opens,

enters and enhances the energy channels of the kidneys and urinary bladder of the human body. Conditions in which improvement can be noted include edema, tinnitus, prostatitis, cystitis, high and low blood pressure, diabetes, nephritis and other renal deficiency problems, gonorrhea, and impotence. In addition, this music also facilitates the weight loss process by breaking down the fatty tissues within the body and improving the metabolism.

PART FIVE

FAQ ABOUT MUSICAL QIGONG

These FAQ (Frequently Asked Questions) are prepared by Shen Wu's Musical Qigong, Inc.

1.   What is Qigong?

Preamble:

•   Internal Organs: According to Chinese medicine, there are five *yin* internal organs and six *yang* internal organs in a human body. The five *yin* organs are the liver, the heart, the spleen (this word in traditional Chinese medicine refers to the digestive system), the lungs, and the kidneys. The six *yang* organs are the gallbladder, the small intestine, the stomach, the large intestine, the urinary bladder, and the triple burner (this is not a physical organ on its own but a functional structure consisting of other organs). Their functions are often more pervasive than those described in Western medicine.

•   Meridians: Meridians are pathways for the movement of Qi within the human body connecting internal organs to other parts of the body. Along the meridians are well-documented points where acupuncturists apply the needling technique to alleviate or cure certain illnesses.

Qigong is a part of traditional Chinese culture that has been practiced for some thousands of years. It is an effective way of promoting health and fitness, as well as developing human potential.

During Qigong training and practice, visualization is of primary importance. The practitioner follows special techniques of visualization, breathing, body gesture and movements, using the energy meridians and pressure points of the body to balance the function of the internal organs with the Qi essence of the universe. This achieves the objectives of cleansing the body and the mind, restoring energy, and opening up the patient's physical and mental potential, thereby strengthening the body mechanism and promoting the circulation and supply of Qi and blood. As a result, Qigong is a very effective self-healing practice for patients with various illnesses.

The objectives of practicing Qigong lie in three main areas: cleansing of the body and the mind, restoration of energy, and development of one's physical and mental potential.

a.   Cleansing of the body and mind:

Special techniques of visualization, breathing, body gesture and movements are used to cleanse and purify the body and the mind. This is the foundation of Qigong training, especially in today's polluted world, where people are emotionally distressed. In this process energy is also gained and stored, and one's potential is further developed. From ancient Chinese wisdom come sayings which indicate that if one can place his or her body and mind in this cleansing state during Qigong practice, he or she will arrive at a *yin-yang* harmony, with meridians free of blockages, and a strengthened immune system. For someone with an illness, this is the point in the self-healing process where bad elements are dispelled.

b.   Restoration of energy:

Energy restoration includes generating and storing energy. During the process of mind and body cleansing, the practitioner also gathers the tiny essential elements from the universe (e.g. Qi, light, sound, and other forms of nature's primary energy), which promote the quantity and quality of his or her internal Qi. This is the point in the self-healing process where the immune system is being strengthened.

c.   Development of physical and mental potential:

Development of physical and mental potential includes the enhancement of natural abilities (e.g. improving athletic performance or increasing one's resistance to electric shock), as well as cultivating extraordinary abilities such as telepathy, psychokinesis, and seeing through concrete wall, etc. In fact, the optimum development of human potential requires that the body and mind be regularly cleansed in order that energy be regenerated and effectively stored.

2. What is the relationship between Qigong and Chinese medicine?

Qigong is a formative part of traditional Chinese culture and has a very close relationship with Chinese medicine. In ancient times, Chinese medicine practitioners and Qigong masters always had substantial knowledge of each other's field of expertise. In fact, there is even a belief that fundamental medical principles of *yin* and *yang*, definition of the internal organs, designation of the meridians, description of Qi and blood, etc., all have their origin in Qigong. Qigong has always shared the same theories as Chinese medicine and the two are inseparable from each other.

3. What is Qi?

According to ancient Chinese philosophy, Qi is the substance in the universe from which all things originate, interbreed, and reproduce. Lao-zi believed that Qi is the most elementary substance making up the whole world. *The Book of Zhou-Yi* states: There was mist between heaven and earth, and everything evolved into existence. *The Yellow Emperor's Internal Classics: Plain Questions* states: Qi condenses and procreation begins. Qi disperses and shapes are formed. Qi disseminates and there is growth and reproduction. When Qi comes to an end, the paradigm shifts. In other words, for all living things, birth, growth, reproduction, and death are manifestations of the action of Qi. Zhuang-zi, another great philosopher, had said this in his book *Knowing North Swim*: A man is born when Qi condenses. When Qi comes apart, he dies. This kind of philosophy has penetrated Chinese medicine and has become the foundation and nucleus of Chinese medical theories. It has also greatly influenced the principles of Qigong theories.

Qi = Vital Energy
by Shen Wu

4. What kinds of illnesses are not appropriate for Qigong healing?

In recent years there have been a large number of demonstrated cases of successful Qigong treatment. As a result, people often assume that one can perform Qigong for self healing of all kinds of diseases. This is, however, a misconception. There are certain diseases where self-healing Qigong treatment should be used with great caution or should not be used at all. For those who have the following illnesses or symptoms Qigong should not be used for self-treatment:

• Certain mental illnesses, such as manic psychosis, and certain schizophrenic diseases. For some other mental illnesses, patients can practice Musical Qigong for self-healing purposes when they are clear-minded.

• Certain acute abdominal syndromes, such as acute suppurative cholecystitis, acute suppurative appendicitis, acute gastrobrosis, acute hemorrhagic pancreatitis, late stage enteremphraxis (intestinal obstruction) and acute appendicitis with diffuse pleurisy. When these syndromes are evident, Qigong practice cannot alleviate the problems.

• Acute cardiemphraxis. One should never self-treat by practicing Musical Qigong when this disease is active. One can practice only after the episode.

• Mania and epilepsy should never be self-treated by practicing Musical Qigong when this disease is active. One can practice only after the episode.

Generally speaking, it is prohibited to use Qigong for treating acute diseases during the acute episode. Only after the disease has slowed down or entered the chronic stage can Qigong be used as self-treatment. Moreover, one should carefully identify the disease pattern and choose the suitable Qigong sets for practice in order to achieve optimal health.

In addition, paralyzed patients and those who cannot get out of bed, as well as those with diseases at a very late and severe stage, should not practice any Qigong. However, anyone can listen to Qigong music for diseases and conditions of all kinds. Since special Qigong messages are incorporated into the music, playing the music is like having the Qigong master perform Qigong treatment for the listener. Therefore, while it is inappropriate to practice Qigong for certain diseases, it is safe and beneficial to listen to Qigong music at any time.

5.   Why can Qigong training heal diseases?

Qigong training teaches the gathering and storing of Primary Qi (good, positive, and life sustaining Qi from the universe), which is the foundation of the entire human body. In ancient times people had created many types of Qigong to keep fit and prolong life, such as Tu Na (special inhale and exhale methods), tai chi, the Five Animal Play, etc. Through adjusting the body, the breathing, and the mind, Qigong training enables the circulation of Primary Qi within the body and enhances the immune response.

6.   Can other kinds of treatment be received by the patient under Qigong training?

Yes. The ancient Chinese medical treatment and the modern Western medicine and treatment are both fruits of laborious scientific exploration on the mystery of human life. Each has its own merits and indispensable usage and should not be considered competing against one another. Qigong treatment may also be complemented by other techniques such as acupuncture, massage, bone correction, herbal medicine intake, etc.

7.   Can Qigong heal all kinds of diseases?

No. Qigong is only one major component of a comprehensive health care program. Just like any other medicine, be it Eastern or Western, Qigong cannot heal all kinds of diseases.

125

Therefore, it is desirable to discover the illness at its earliest stage, have it treated, and practice Qigong diligently. Also, it is always better to prevent than to heal using Qigong practice.

8.   How was Shen Wu's Musical Qigong founded?

Master Shen Wu combined ancient medical theories together with the five notes. With passion, hard work, and experimentation, he founded the world's first Qigong style that combines modern music and Qigong. As a result, Shen Wu's Musical Qigong (Dong Fang Fu Yin Gong in Chinese) has been tested and approved by the Chinese Qigong Science Research Institute as a top rated, modern Qigong style.

9.   What are the theories behind Shen Wu's Musical Qigong?

Shen Wu's Musical Qigong is based on the principle of the five notes corresponding to the five *yin* organs. Using sound waves as the medium, the energy is transferred via skin pores to affect the internal organs. The special sonic energy combines with Qigong signals (hidden messages) and acts as a massive force of energy flow. It promotes the Qi and blood circulation within the body and expels the disease-causing (bad and evil) Qi, resulting in strengthening one's body and mind and promoting recovery from illnesses.

10.   How is Shen Wu's Musical Qigong different from other Qigong styles?

Shen Wu's Musical Qigong combines the benefits of music and Qigong, which distinguishes itself among other non-music Qigong styles. Specially arranged musical rhythms and melodies constitute a great sound wave energy source. When this energy is overlaid with Qigong energy, the resultant energy vector exhibits a "1 + 1 > 2" phenomenon, meaning an energy reinforcement with a greater than proportionate magnitude. It is thus more effective in promoting Qi and blood circulation, expelling disease-causing Qi, and enhancing body and mind.

Shen Wu's Musical Qigong contains very simple movement sets. It uses the "music thoughts" to replace thousands of "stray thoughts" (worries, anxiety, fear, distrust, etc.). It is not confined by any factors such as time, space, location, cultural level, body constitution, etc.

However, Shen Wu's Musical Qigong does not pose any conflict with other Qigong styles. Rather, it constitutes a complimentary and beneficial relationship. As a result, Shen Wu's Musical Qigong is highly suitable for modern people from all walks of life with a wide variety of working tempos.

11. Why should we listen to different Qigong music for treating different illnesses?

According to the principles of correspondence between the five elements, the five notes, and the five *yin* organs in the body, specific Qigong music (sound and rhythm) corresponds to specific internal organs and meridians. Therefore, based on the location of the problem area in the body, one may choose the Qigong music, targeting that area through the meridians to balance the body and the mind in order to yield the optimum treatment results. The five notes of Qigong music treat problems corresponding to the five *yin* and *yang* organs. The five CDs in the "Life Music for Healing" series harmonize and regulate the whole body. Cancer patients should listen to all of them.

12. Why do the audio and video tapes of Shen Wu's Musical Qigong have healing power?

It is because Master Shen Wu im-
bedded the energy of the sound waves
directly into the Qigong messages
during the production of these video
and audio tapes.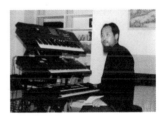

13.   Can pregnant women listen to Shen Wu's Musical Qigong tapes and CDs?

Yes. These Qigong tapes and CDs can adjust the Qi and blood condition for pregnant women and the fetus, promoting an excellent development for the fetus and increasing the elasticity of its cerebral cortex, so that a more intelligent and healthy baby will be born. For purposes of subliminal fetal training for excellence, the pregnant woman, while listening to the tape, can nonchalantly suggest with her mind that the baby will be very healthy and intelligent. However, it is extremely important to remember that pregnant women should not practice movement (dynamic) Qigong. Nor should they do any mental concentration on any part of the body either.

14.   What are the benefits for the students who listen to Shen Wu's Qigong music?

The music can strengthen the bio-magnetic field of the brain, improve memory significantly, enhance elasticity of the cerebral cortex, reduce mental fatigue, and increase intelligence. It can also improve students psyche, help remove pre-examination panic as well as nervousness and temporary forgetfulness during examinations, resulting in better grades and a happier school life.

15.   How much time should be spent each day listening to Qigong music tapes and practicing movement Qigong?

One should listen to Qigong music and practice quiescent Qigong for not less than sixty minutes each day. One should practice movement Qigong for at least 30 minutes each day. The four best times to practice Qigong are 5-7 a.m., 11 a.m.-1 p.m., 5-7 p.m., and 11 p.m.-1 a.m. It is during these times that the north-south magnetic field of the earth is the strongest, and the effect of the electromagnetic field and radiation is the strongest. For children, the best results come from listening to Qigong music during their sleep.

16. What kinds of illnesses can be effectively treated by Shen Wu's Musical Qigong tapes?

It is most effective for treating diseases caused by functional imbalances of the nervous system, respiratory system, circulatory system, endocrine system, and digestive system.

It also effectively treats gynecological diseases as well as diseases associated with the five sensory organs. These diseases include: neurasthenia, sciatica, hemiplegia, migraine, upper track infection, chronic bronchitis, pulmonary emphysema, asthma, pulmonary tuberculosis, angina pectoris, cardiac arrhythmia, arteriosclerosis, hypertension, hypotension, thrombosis, diabetes mellitus, gall stones, nephritis, nephrasthenia, gastritis, hepatitis-B, numbness of the four limbs, rheumatoid arthritis, bone growth, splintered fracture, lumbar and leg pain, hysteromyoma, breast gland growth, banal breast tumor, myopia, deafness, rhinitis, glaucoma, etc.

Because the treatment principles of Shen Wu's Musical Qigong are rather different from those of western medicine, it is usually very effective in treating obscure and difficult cases that western medicine is powerless about.

17. Is Shen Wu's Qigong music still effective when the listener falls asleep?

Yes. When one enters sleep mode, although his or her consciousness is at rest, the Qigong embedded in the musical sound wave is still working on his or her body. Through the skin pores into the meridians and internal organs, Qigong music is effective in restoring, working and enhancing the functioning of the cerebrum and the internal organs.

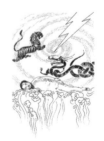

18. What is the best way to listen to Shen Wu's Qigong music to get better treatment results?

It is necessary to adjust oneself to enter the Qi-receiving state. Relax the whole body, and arrive at a peaceful, quiet, and natural state. Regulate one's breathing. Replace the thousands of thoughts with one thought — the music thought.

After listening to the Qigong music, remember to perform the "closing" routine. Rub both hands together so that the palms are warm or hot. Place both palms, one on top of the other, on the lower *Dantian* area (lower abdomen). Deeply and slowly, take three breaths into the lungs. When exhaling, lower the Qi from the lungs into the lower *Dantian* area (mostly by visualization). By doing this, one can obtain the maximum benefits from listening to the Qigong music.

19. Why is it that patients without the intent of being treated can still be positively treated while listening to the Qigong music?

Whether one has the intent or not, sound waves carrying Shen Wu's Qigong energy and messages can still work on him or her, regulating the whole body and the mind in a beneficial way.

20. Why is it beneficial to practice vegetarianism during Qigong training?

The internal organs of a vegetarian are well cleansed, allowing him or her to be more grounded and focused during meditation. Eating meat can cause heavier breathing by the nose and mouth, making it more difficult to adjust one's breathing for quiescent Qigong practice. Also, eating spicy food can cause Qi to disperse and become deficient. Therefore, Qigong practitioners should avoid spicy food.

During Qigong practice, there may be a time when a Qigong

practitioner feels like being vegetarian. It is normal because his or her body is probably signaling a need for cleansing. When that happens, just allow it to happen naturally. After a while, some practitioners may go back to eating both meat and vegetables while others may remain a vegetarian for a longer time, or forever, depending on one's biological needs. Do not force this issue. Everything should be done naturally according its own course.

21.   What is the meridian network?

The Meridian Network, pronounced as *Jing Luo* in Chinese, is a sophisticated and weblike roadway for the movement and circulation of internal bodily Qi. It is made up of *Jing* meridians (main channels) and *Luo* meridians (collateral channels) crisscrossing each other within the body, connecting all internal organs with each other and to all parts of the body. An unobstructed circulation of Qi within the meridian network promotes blood circulation, aids in the balance of *yin* and *yang*, and enhances the healthy development of internal organs as well as bone and joint structures. It also facilitates the harmony between internal energy and our living environment, enabling us to lead a happy and healthy life.

Jing meridians in the body are like rivers — straight, deep, long and big; they are the main flows of the meridian network. *Luo* meridians in the body are like a hunting net — spanning sideways, shallow, short and small; they are the tributaries of the *Jing* meridians, connecting them and allowing a complete circulatory pathway for Qi and blood.

When Qi and blood are traveling along the *Jing Luo* meridians unobstructed, the body enjoys a balanced state of *yin* and *yang*, which means a good health. When Qi and blood are somehow obstructed while moving along the *Jing Luo* meridians, illnesses arise.

When practicing Qigong, one may guide the movement of internal Qi to circulate along set routes of *Jing* and *Luo* meridians. The purpose is to prevent and open up any blockages of the meridians and to ensure unobstructed movement of Qi and blood throughout various internal organs and the rest of the body.

Along the *Jing Luo* meridians, there are various locations where the Qi and blood of the internal organs gather and collect. They are called the *Xue* points (acupunture points or acupoints).

22.   How many Jing Luo meridians are there in the body?

The body contains twelve regular *Jing Luo* Meridians and eight extra-meridians. Qi and blood circulate in the body along the meridians in the following order:

1. the Lung Meridian,

2. the Large Intestine Meridian,

3. the Stomach Meridian,

4. the Spleen Meridian,

5. the Heart Meridian,

6. the Small Intestine Meridian,

7. the Urinary Bladder Meridian,

8. the Kidney Meridian,

9. the Pericardium Meridian,

10. the Triple Burner Meridian,

11. the Gallbladder Meridian,

12. the Liver Meridian,

and then back to the Lung Meridian. Meridians of *yin* organs

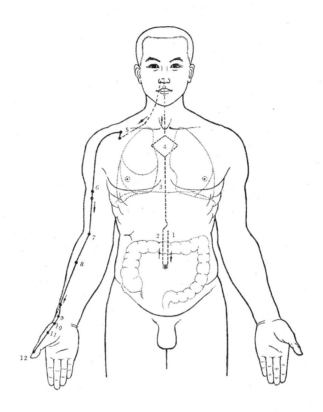

*Qi and blood movement
along the 12 regular Jing Luo Meridians*

are called *yin* meridians and those of *yang* organs are called *yang* meridians.

The eight extra meridians are so called because they do not connect directly to internal organs and, except for the *Ren* and *Du* meridians, they do not contain any acupuncture points. Situated between the regular meridians, the extra-meridians regulate the Qi and blood of the regular meridians. In Qigong practice, three of these extra meridians (*Du* Meridian, *Ren* Merid-

133

ian, and *Dai* Meridian) are especially important. The *Du* Meridian begins in the front abdominal area, and flows down to the perineum, up all the way along the spine, up and over the top of the head and down the forehead to below the nose. It has the function of governing all the *yang* meridians in the body. *Ren* Meridian begins in the pelvic cavity, emerges at the perineum, goes up the front (along centerline) all the way passing the throat, the chin, circumventing the lips and up through the cheeks into the eyes. It has the functions of governing all the *yin* meridians in the body. (For illustrations, see Page 66). *Dai* Meridian, also called the *Belt* Meridian, is situated around the waist like a belt.

23. What kind of Jing Luo meridian sensation would Qigong practice bring about?

When practicing Qigong, one may feel sensations of heat, swelling, tickling, etc. in certain parts of the body. One may also feel a warm current flowing along a certain path within the body. This is the manifestation of internal Qi movement along the *Jing Luo* meridians.

APPENDIX

I

CASES AND TESTIMONIALS

Master Shen Wu has treated thousands of patients since he came to the United States in mid 1990s. These people, coming from all parts of the world, range from chronic pain sufferers to terminal cancer patients. Here you will see some cases and hear what the patients have said about Master Wu and his Musical Qigong treatment.

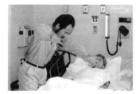 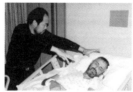 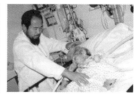

■ Brain Cancer Patient Artreis Dobbins

Mrs. Artreis Dobbins had chemotherapy and radiation for lung cancer in 1997, was discovered to have brain cancer in 1998, and was diagnosed to have 3 tumors in 1999. She had been receiving Master Wu's treatment regularly each week since March 1999. Her general condition had improved a great deal. She no longer complained of pain, slept better, and had 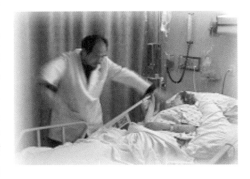 a good appetite. She also began socializing and going places again.

"Ms. Dobbins was seen in my office. She has undergone extensive work up. She has had a bone scan on June 11 which showed abnormal uptake in the left lower ribs, right ribs and right femoral neck. CT scan of the chest showed a comma-shaped density and questionable cavitary lesion. MRI brain in May 1999 showed marked improvement in the tumor in the brain in the right frontal masses to be proved. At the present time, she has elected not to have any chemotherapy. She is to continue her care with you (Master Wu)."

— Dr. Thomas J. Katta, M.D., Winter Park Memorial Hospital, Orlando, Florida

MRI Reports on Mrs. Dobbins' Diseases

The first MRI report on Mrs. Dobbins showed two tumors had disappeared. It was May 1999. The second MRI taken in September 1999 showed that a small area of edema in the right frontal lobe was significantly smaller than previous study. No pathologic contrast enhancement was identified. No new pathology was noted in the interval.

These MRI reports have been verified by Dr. Thomas
Katta of Winter Park Memorial Hospital, Orlando, Florida.

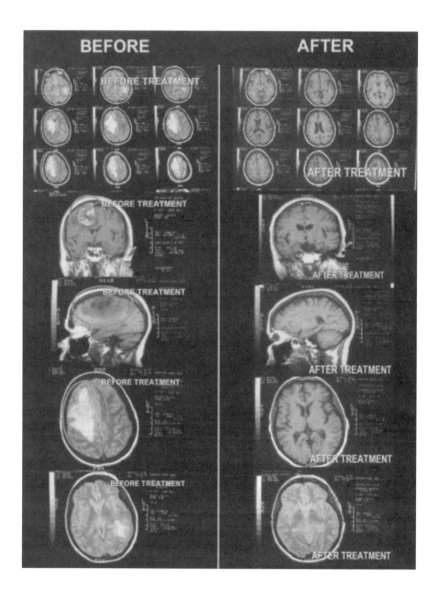

■ Breast Cancer Patient Carol Smith

"What Master Wu has done for me cannot be explained in words. It can only be felt within ... and then, by the outside result, one can see for themselves the 'gift of the man.' Master Wu is truly a uniquely, gifted man and has been blessed with many talents. His is a purpose not understood by many, yet hoped for by all. Not only did he share with me the 'Gift of Healing,' but he also shared a rare kind of wisdom that was stored not by the mind but within each minute particle of my being. I felt it 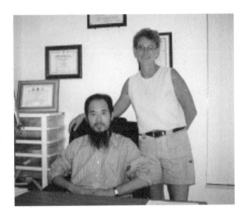 deeper with each treatment that I had. It was a gift that was given with a pure heart and a noble spirit.

After a long journey and much intense work, it was a joy for me to find someone who truly cared for me as an individual and shared his gift of energy therapy with such tenacity, kindness and love. The gift of healing that was given unto me through Master Wu is, and continues to be, a 'blessing fulfilled' as each day passes.

Rare is the man who gives without expecting a thing in return but a smile upon the face of the one who graces his domain. Master Wu is such a man. And as they say, behind every great man stands an honorable woman. Together, the combination of the two touches lives in such a way that one shall never remain the same but will move forward in newness, health and growth. That's the way you feel after having met and spent time with Master Wu.

Master Wu is to be commended for his contribution not only to each of us individually, but to all mankind.

My highest regards to Master Wu for being a healer of such great magnitude and a teacher to be proud of. He is one of the few who lives his truth and for that, he continues to be Blessed in all that he does and through those whose lives he touches."

■ **Liver Disease Patient Eliza Mao**

Eliza Mao is a registered nurse who had worked for the Federal Government for more than 11 years. She went to see Master Wu for an alternative treatment after all conventional treatments had failed for her liver disease.

"I found myself getting stronger physically and better emotionally each day, and practice Qigong daily and realize how important Qigong is to human body. I decided to follow Master Wu's footstep to teach people the theory and exercise of Qigong, to bring back good health to people."

Eliza left her government job in California and relocated to Florida in September 1997, to work on trial program of cancer pain control with Dr. N. Finkler (center) and Master Wu.

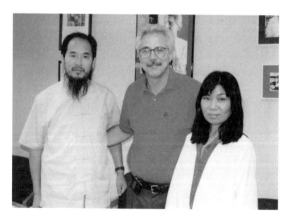

■ **Kidney Infection Patient Victor**

"I am writing this letter as a reference to Master Shen Wu's special ability to treat patients. My name is Wesley Kwan, I am

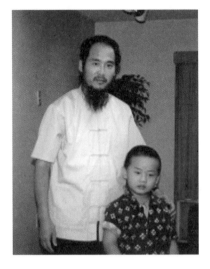

registered pharmacist in the state of Florida and state of Maryland. My 4 year-old son, Victor, went to a routine physical exam and found out that his urine contained blood and protein and he has been diagnosed with a kidney infection. Under strong recommendation, we decided to let him try Master Shen Wu's 'Qi Treatment.' He treats him with 'Qi Treatment' without giving him any medication. After 5 days we send him to SKB lab to do the test again. Like magic, this time the test result came up all negative.

I have been practicing pharmacy for more than 20 years and I always believe in the trust of Western medicine. This to me is totally unheard of; the only explanation is that Master Wu's special ability and his 'Qi Treatment' are really become a nice alternative and new dimension for health science."

Wesley Kwan

■ Endometrial Cancer Patient Gini W. Cucuel

"I have come to know Shen Wu and value him as a Master of Qigong and the Founder of Dong Fang Fu Yin Musical Qigong. From my experience with Master Wu I can declare that his musical Qigong alignment and balancing sessions, as well as his ability to train others in Qigong thought and practice, are assets of considerable benefit to the citizens of the United States. He has taught me and many other persons how to regain health and physical, mental, emotional and spiritual fitness.

141

Master Wu's dedication to his calling and to his clients goes far beyond what might be expected. He provides a healthful alternative for persons seeking an adjunct to western medical thought and practice. For him to be able to continue his work in this country will be of benefit to a wide variety of people who seek his help with medical and personal crises.

After a diagnosis of endometrial cancer and a host of other physical disabilities, I have been restored to considerable health and a marvelous sense of well-being as a direct result of consulting with Master Wu. I have met several other persons who experience a far superior quality of life than they had thought possible since entering treatment and training with Master Wu. He has a collection of "before and after" tests done by American doctors indicating the positive treatment effects of Master 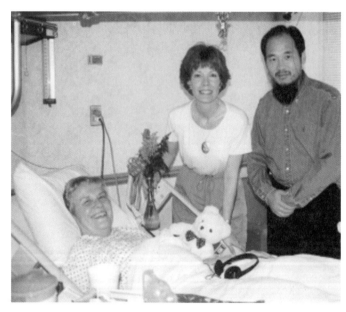 Wu's Musical Qigong. As a lifelong citizen of the United States of America, I feel that we Americans are honored to have a person of Master Wu's credentials and caliber in this country."

■ Parkinson's Disease Patient Henry Leung

Mr. Henry Leung, 70 and suffering from Parkinson's disease for 28 years, as well as hypertension and kidney problem, had 2 months of Musical Qigong therapy last year and was taught to do Musical Qigong exercise. This year Mr. Henry Leung has been treated since the 31st of January. Mrs. Leung said her husband's condition has improved a great deal from grade 3 to grade 2.

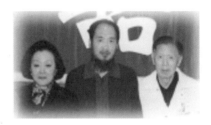

■ "Master Wu has given me a second lease on life."

Leandro Larrosa, severe internal injury sufferer

Famous international racer and multi-champion, who suffered severe internal injuries from a car accident. Following 10 treatments by Master Wu, Larrosa recovered fully.

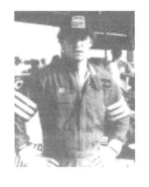

■ "Master Wu is a remarkable genius in a new field of medicine – use of resonant music coupled with Qigong. I think I have improved sufficiently that I am confident, with the grace of God... I will make it."

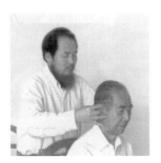

Lawrence Jue, hearing impaired patient

Mechanical Engineer, P. E., U.S. Naval Architect

■ **"The result was extraordinary!"**

Chet Jaworski, chronic aches and pains sufferer

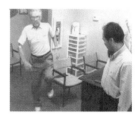

Basketball legend, Class of 1939, the first URI All-American and the national scoring champion

■ **"After the workshop, Master Wu gave me two short treatments, which quickly and dramatically reduced the pain in my shoulder, and I was able to resume playing the violin immediately ... I truly appreciate Master Wu's exceptional gift of healing and I feel privileged and fortunate to have met him."**

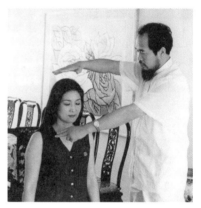

Ling Ling Guan, shoulder pain sufferer

Violinist at the St. Louis Symphony Orchestra

■ **"I love Master Wu's music. The rich variety of melodious tunes in his music makes me feel extremely relaxed."**

Anna, cancer patient

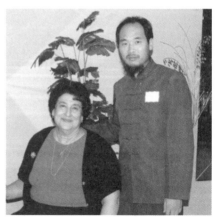

Pianist, who, after receiving 17 Musical Qigong treatments from Master Wu, felt her life had greatly changed. She regarded herself as a healthy person again.

144

■ Susan's Story

"I would not be alive without Master Wu!"

Susan Chang, Pancreatic Tumor Patient

In June 2000, Susan Chang of New Jersey was diagnosed with pancreatic tumor. All of her doctors said that she needed immediate surgery. The news was so devastating to her that she felt her life was over. She was very reluctant to take the surgery, afraid that she might not come out of the operation room alive, and never being able 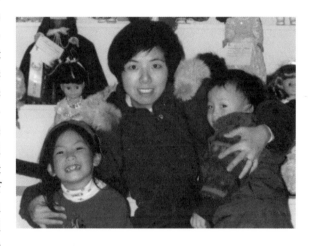 to see her husband and two small children again. She told herself that Master Shen Wu was her only hope.

She came to see Master Wu in July 2000 and after two months' treatments (without any other kind of therapy), the CT scan and all the tests showed that her tumor had dissolved. Her recovery is truly amazing and she feels that she has been given a second life.

Now, the Qigong exercises, along with listening to the music of Master Wu's CDs, have become a daily ritual for her. She is eternally grateful to Master Wu for his healing power. Without seeking his treatment, Susan Chang feels she would not be alive today.

II

HONORS AND AWARDS

Master Shen Wu has been awarded many prizes and honors and he has appeared, among others, on NBC, CBS and TBS. Master Wu has also been interviewed by major Chinese media as North American Chinese Television Stations, New York Chinese Television Station and Hong Kong Star Television. Extensive coverage on Master Shen Wu and his Musical Qigong has appeared in World Journal, Orlando Weekly, China Qigong Science, International News, U.S. Digest and Washington News.

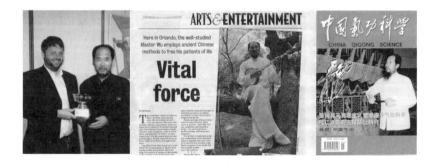

MUSICAL QIGONG

To appreciate and honor what Master Shen Wu had done to promote the cultural exchange between East and West, President Bill Clinton and members of the Congress met Master Wu in New York on April 25, 2000, during which the President also congratulated Master Wu on his receiving the Cannes Festival 2000 -- Asian Cutlure Exhibition award for his documentary "Music before Medicine."

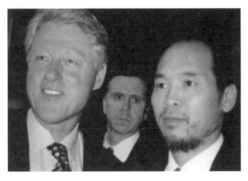

Master Shen Wu with President Bill Clinton

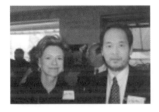

Congresswoman Judith Hope

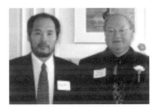

Congressman Gary Ackerman

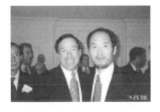

Congressman Steve Forbes

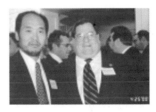

Congressman Jerrold Nadler

Letter from the First Lady of Hawaii to Master Shen Wu thanking him for his music and his tireless work in Musical Qigong therapy.

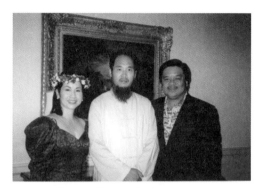

Master Wu with Governor and First Lady of Hawaii

April 23, 1999

Dear Master Wu:

Thank you for sharing the video on your supernatural power of healing. Your unique treatment for pain control and healing is miraculous and very inspirational. I am very interested in sharing with close relatives and friends how this alternative therapy can enhance one's quality of life and would like to obtain some additional copies if they are available. Your therapy brings much hope especially to those who have exhausted all the recommended medical options. It is a blessing to have learned about your special treatment.

With warmest personal regards,

Vicky T Cayetano

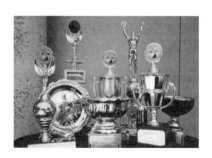

Part of the honors, prizes and awards Master Wu has received for his Musical Qigong therapy.

RESEARCH AND ACADEMIC EXCHANGE

Currently Master Shen Wu is working closely with Dr. Neil J. Finkler at Walt Disney Memorial Cancer Institute, and Dr. Thomas J. Katta of Winter Park Memorial Hospital, both traditional medical oncologists in the Orlando area, regarding various treatments for their late stage cancer patients. Master Shen Wu is also cooperating with Dr. Mehmet C. Oz, Assistant Professor of Surgery at Columbia University's College of Physicians & Surgeons, for development on alternative medicine.

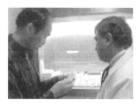
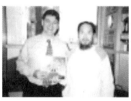
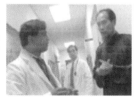

■ Cancer Trial Program

"During the calendar year 1998 and early 1999, the division of gynecologic oncology at the Walt Disney Memorial Cancer Institute at Florida Hospital collaborated with Master Wu in a nonrandomized, uncontrolled trial on evaluating the effects of Qigong therapy in patients with end-stage cancer and pain. The purpose of this short-term trial was to evaluate whether Qigong therapy had any beneficial effects with regards to reducing pain associated with terminal pelvic cancer. Approximately 15 patients were enrolled in this trial and underwent Qigong therapy with Master Wu on an as-needed basis in an attempt to reduce narcotics requirements associated with their terminal malignancy. During the course of this trial, it became quite apparent that all of the patients studied had marked reduction in their narcotic requirement. In several patients, narcotics were able to be discontinued totally and pain relief continued with Qigong therapy alone. Although this was a nonrandomized, uncontrolled trial, it is interesting to note that the life expectancy of the majority of patients with terminal malignancies turned out to be far greater than one would have expected with standard conventional therapies alone.

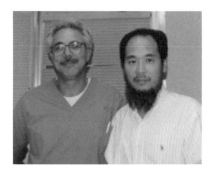

The study showed such promising effects of Qigong therapy that we are presently planning a large-scale prospectively controlled trial in an effort to try to reproduce these results on a larger scale."

— Dr. Neil J. Finkler, M.D., Walt Disney Memorial Cancer Institute Florida Hospital

■ **Comprehensive Cancer Care 2000 Conference**

Master Shen Wu was invited to attend Comprehensive Cancer Care 2000 Conference (CCC 2000) from June 9-11 in the Greater Washington D.C. area. The goal for CCC 2000 is to bring those who are conducting the most innovative research on complementary and alternative therapies for cancer together with the most distinguished mainstream oncologists to evaluate promising therapies and how they can successfully be integrated into comprehensive cancer care.

• Master Wu with Mr. Stephen E. Straus, M.D., Director of the National Center for Complementary and Alternative Medicine of the National Institutes of Health. Dr. Straus attaches great importance to Master Wu's Musical Qigong 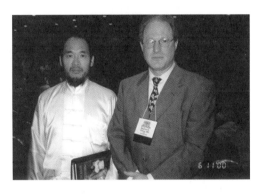 therapy and he really loves the idea of "music before medicine." He said: "We have a lot to learn from Master Wu."

• With Ms. Elda Railey, Director of Grants and Sponsored Programs for the Susan G. Komen Breast Cancer Foundation. Ms. Railey is very impressed by Master Wu's cancer research and treatment programs and encourages him to apply for their grant.

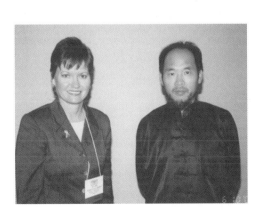

151

• With Dr. David Ringer of American Cancer Society (left) and Dr. Phuong Thi Kim Pham, Program Director at the National Cancer Institute (center).

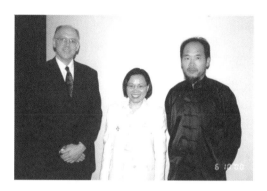

• The Honorable Berkley Bedell, Congressman of 6 terms and Founder and President of the National Foundation for Alternative Medicine (right) and Jeffrey White, M.D., Director of Office of Cancer Complementary and Alternative Medicine at the National Cancer Institute (left) are very impressed and interested with Master Shen Wu's achievements. They strongly support Dr. Finkler to continue working with Master Wu for further research.

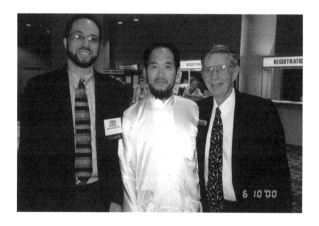

Index

PRODUCTS FROM
SHEN WU MUSICAL QIGONG, INC.

Compact Disks

SHINING SPRING

Wood Music for Liver

By Shen Wu, $20

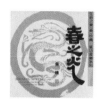

RECEPTIVE SOULS

Fire Music for Heart

By Shen Wu, $20

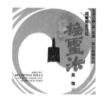

A JOURNEY

IN HARMONY I

Earth Music for Spleen

By Shen Wu, $20

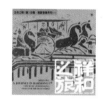

HEAVENLY TUNES

Metal Music for Lungs

By Shen Wu, $20

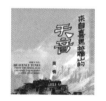

A JOURNEY

IN HARMONY II

Water Music for Kidneys

By Shen Wu, $20

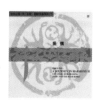

**Musical Qigong
Therapeutic
Collections
by Shen Wu
Set of 5 Audio Tapes
$80.00 / set**

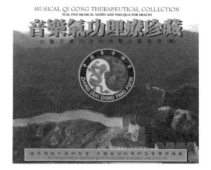

**Musical Qigong
Demonstration
Vedio Tapes
by Shen Wu
$100.00 / Tape**

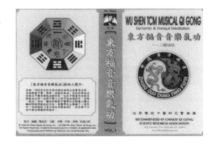

**The Making of
Musical Qigong &
A Biography of
Shen Wu
(in Chinese)
$35.00**

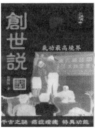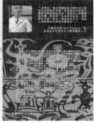

www.homabooks.com
More titles from Homa & Sekey Books

Flower Terror: Suffocating Stories of China
by Pu Ning, ISBN 0-9665421-0-X
Autobiographical Stories, Paperback, $13.95

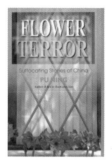

Acclaimed Chinese writer eloquently describes the oppression of intellectuals in his country between 1950s and 1970s in these twelve autobiographical novellas and short stories. Many of the stories are so shocking and heart-wrenching that one cannot but feel suffocated.

"The stories in this work are well written." — *Library Journal*

The Peony Pavilion: A Novel by Xiaoping Yen
ISBN 0-9665421-2-6, Fiction, Paperback, $16.95

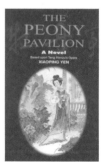

A sixteen-year-old girl visits a forbidden garden and falls in love with a young man she meets in a dream. She has an affair with her dreamlover and dies longing for him. After her death, her unflagging spirit continues to wait for her dreamlover. Does her lover really exist? Can a youthful love born of a garden dream ever blossom?

Based on a famous sixteenth-century Chinese opera written by Tang Xianzu, "the Shakespeare of China," the novel leads the reader into a mythical world of passion and romance. Its many fascinating characters include a failed scholar, a Taoist nun, a husband and wife rebel team, a dissolute emperor, and Tartar invaders from the North.

"A window into the Chinese literary imagination." — *Publishers Weekly*

Butterfly Lovers: A Tale of the Chinese Romeo and Juliet
by Fan Dai, ISBN 0-9665421-4-2, Paperback, $16.95

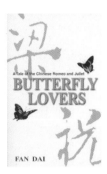

A beautiful girl disguises herself as a man and lives under one roof with a young male scholar for three years without revealing her true identity. They become sworn brothers, soul mates and lovers. In a world in which marriage is determined by social status and arranged by parents, what is their inescapable fate? The novel is based upon a popular Chinese story of forbidden love that has moved millions to tears.

"An engaging, compelling, deeply moving, highly recommended and rewarding novel." — *Midwest Book Review*

Always Bright: Paintings by American Chinese Artists 1970-1999
Edited by Henry Riseman, Xue Jian Xin et al.
ISBN 0-9665421-3-4, Art, Hardcover, $49.95

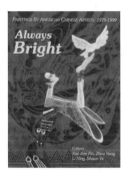

Selected paintings by eighty acclaimed American Chinese artists in the late twentieth century, *Always Bright* falls into three categories: oil painting, Chinese painting and other media painting. With profiles of the artists and information on their professional accomplishment, the book fills a blank in the American Chinese art book publication and satisfies an increasing need from readers who crane to know American Chinese artists and their art.

Order Information
Please send a check or money order (payable to Homa & Sekey Books) for each ordered book plus $3.50 shipping & handling to: Orders Department, Homa & Sekey Books, 138 Veterans Plaza, P.O. Box 103, Dumont, NJ 07628.